Eat Your Greens

The Channel 4 television series *Grow Your Greens*
and *Eat Your Greens* was produced by
Wall to Wall Television.

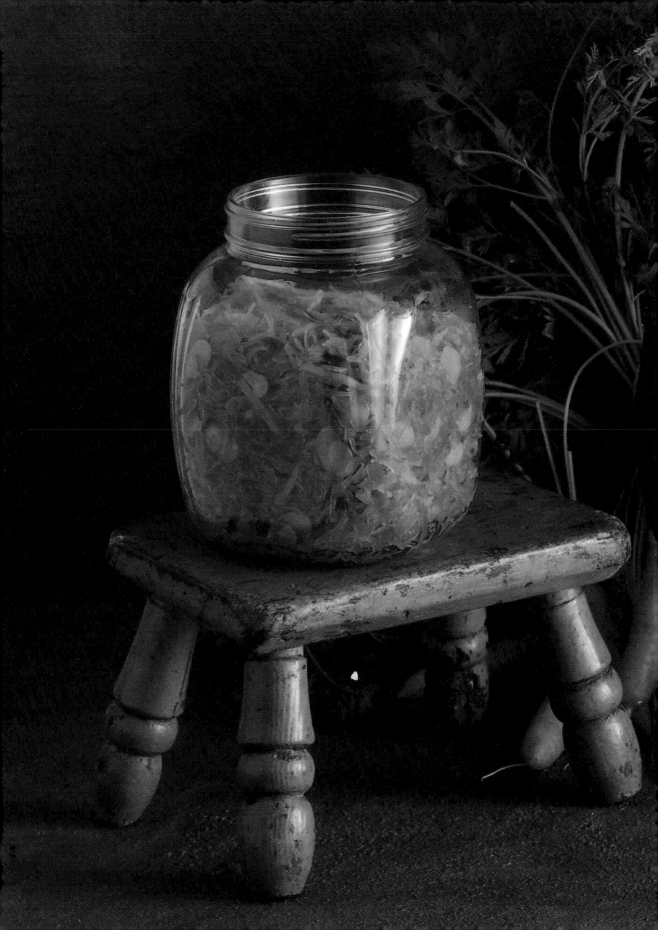

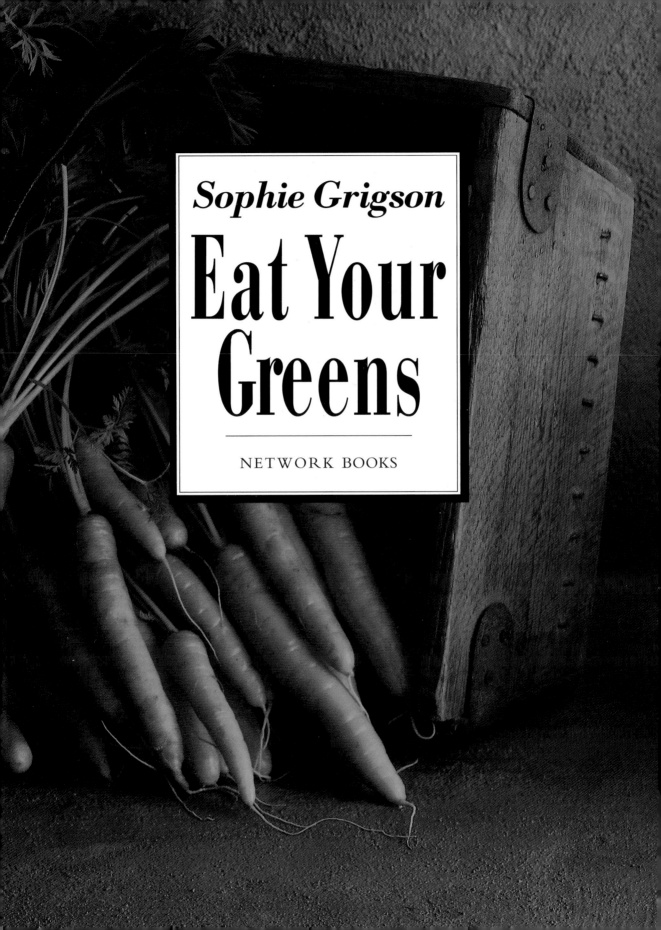

Sophie Grigson

Eat Your Greens

NETWORK BOOKS

For William
who has made me happier than I ever thought possible

Network Books is an imprint of BBC Books,
a division of BBC Enterprises Limited
Woodlands, 80 Wood Lane, London W12 0TT
First published 1993

© Sophie Grigson 1993
The moral right of the author has been asserted
ISBN 0 563 36738 5

Designed by Tim Higgins
Illustrations © Linda Smith
Photographs by Jess Koppel
Styling by Roisin Nield
Home Economist: Lyn Rutherford

The author and publisher would like to thank the following
for permission to reproduce copyright material.
JOHN TOVEY'S LIGHTLY CURRIED, DEEP-FRIED CELERY STRIPS,
© John Tovey from *Feast of Vegetables*, Century, 1985
PAJON © Mark and Kim Millon from *The Flavours of Korea*, André
Deutsch, 1991
MEFARKA and CLAUDIA RODEN'S SWEET AUBERGINE PRESERVE © Claudia
Roden from *New Book of Middle Eastern Food*, Penguin, 1986
BRIGID ALLEN'S GREEN VELVET SOUP and BRIGID ALLEN'S BROAD BEAN
SOUP WITH PESTO © Brigid Allen, from *The Soup Book*, Papermac, 1993
JOYCE MOLYNEUX'S ONION AND SOURED CREAM SALAD,
© Joyce Molyneux from *The Carved Angel Cookery Book*
(with Sophie Grigson), Grafton, 1992

Set in Monotype Bodoni Bold and Bembo by
Ace Filmsetting Ltd, Frome, Somerset
Printed in Great Britain by Cambus Litho Ltd, East Kilbride
Bound in Great Britain by Charles Letts Ltd, Edinburgh
Colour separations by Technik, Berkhamsted, Herts
Jacket printed by Belmont Press, Northampton

TITLE PAGE *Oded Schwartz's Carrot and Almond Chutney*

Contents

Acknowledgements

I have my mother to thank, first and foremost, for my love of vegetables. She cooked them perfectly and lovingly and imaginatively. I don't ever remember disliking vegetables, as so many children did. My most used cookery book is still my mother's *Vegetable Book*, by far the best book ever written on the subject. I would never have dreamed of writing a book on vegetables myself if it hadn't been for Sue Shepherd of Channel 4 and Jane Root and Joanne Reay of Wall to Wall Television. When they asked me to present a television series on vegetables I was thrilled, and this book was the natural follow-on.

Filming and writing the book simultaneously has sometimes been tough going. Everyone at Wall to Wall has been tremendously supportive, but I would particularly like to thank the two directors, Basil Comely and Alexa Marengo for all their encouragement and patience with a novice presenter, and the two marvellous researchers, Patricia Llewellyn and Helen Fletcher, who unearthed a remarkable collection of contributors. Jack Sainte-Rose and Toria Russell have kept everything running smoothly throughout. And thanks must go, too, to Joy Larcom who has helped with so many gardening queries.

I've been lucky to have calm, constructive but not interfering editors, Heather Holden-Brown and Deborah Taylor of BBC Books, who always believed that I could deliver the manuscript on time, even when I wasn't so sure myself. Sheila Keating, who helped me put the book together and work out how it should be written, has been a tower of strength. I was delighted but not surprised that BBC Books agreed so readily to my first choice of photographer. Jess Koppel's photographs of food prepared by stylist Lyn Rutherford are always a joy to the eye.

Back on the home ranch, I have Annabel Hartog to thank for testing so many recipes so patiently. Most of all I would like to thank my husband, William Black, for marrying me when he knew that I was about to disappear into months of frenzied work, for putting up with my frequent absences, and for always being there when I returned.

Introduction

Who would have expected to find a windswept field of globe artichokes at the end of the wild and beautiful Beara Peninsula in County Cork, Ireland? Or a burgeoning carrot patch at the foot of a lighthouse miles out into the sea off the Isle of Skye? Or a small forest of exotic cardoons amongst the acres of caravans that surround Skegness is a bizarre sight, indeed, but no less so than an extraordinary collection of more than 20 different radishes in an allotment in Shrewsbury. In Kent I met a pea-growing 15-year-old with an immaculately neat allotment, then travelled to Bath to visit an 86-year-old courgette-grower who has worked the same patch of land for 75 years.

The nationwide passion for growing vegetables knows no bounds. It sweeps blithely across all barriers of class, age, religion and race. And it is a passion, there's no doubt about that. While writing this book I've visited gardens, allotments, potagers and odd patches of ground throughout the country, all tended with endless

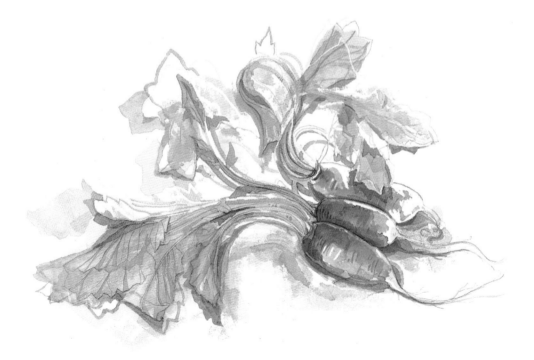

devotion, all yielding bountiful harvests. It's been a summer of unparalleled vegetable delights, infectious enthusiasm and marvellous surprises.

Vegetable growers are generous to a fault. I've returned home time and again clutching bags of freshly picked vegetables with intense flavours that no shop-bought vegetables can hope to match. Home-grown vegetables are an incomparable luxury. I'm green with envy, if you'll excuse the pun, having no more than a handkerchief garden and two cats that grub up every seedling as though it were planted entirely for their personal pleasure.

What perplexes me is that the passion for vegetables seems to end as they come through the kitchen door. This is not entirely true, to be fair. Most of the growers I've met enjoy eating their vegetables almost as much as they enjoy growing them. But as a nation vegetable cookery is not our forte. The 'meat and two veg' ethos still has a strong grip, and it is the meat that stars, while the vegetables are an afterthought cooked with scant attention. Being 'good for you' appears to be their only virtue, and not a particularly appealing one when they are scandalously over-cooked. What a horrible waste! And how depressingly shortsighted and unimaginative.

Even if we can't all enjoy the perfection of home-grown vegetables, we still have a remarkable choice from the greengrocers and supermarkets. There's an enormous and exciting range of tastes, textures and colours in the vegetable realm, from tender greens to orange squashes, floury potatoes to smooth nutty artichokes, bitter chicory to sweet green peas. Meat is really pretty limited in comparison.

As you may well have guessed, I love my vegetables. I love cooking them and I love eating the results even more. Vegetables offer an infinite spectrum of possibilities to the cook. The starting point is learning to treat them with respect, learning to cook them simply to bring out their best. Steaming is my preferred method of plain cooking in most instances as little of the natural flavour is lost to the water. Microwaving works well for many vegetables for the same reason. Over-cooking is the greatest sin, but that doesn't mean that they should be half-raw either. The term *al dente* means tender but still with a slight firmness and resistance as your teeth sink into the centre, and that's what should be aimed for with most vegetables. If they were in good shape, fresh and sprightly in the first place, then attentive cooking and a knob of butter melting over them in the serving dish will show them off at their purest.

One shouldn't become too obsessed with *al dente*-ism though. It is not always what's called for. Potatoes are an obvious exception, but there are others, such as pumpkin or squashes which need to be cooked to a melting softness. Many of the brassicas, from cabbage through to broccoli, take on a whole new persona when slowly, lengthily braised in their own juices, butter or oil, and little or no water.

In this book, I've gathered together some of my favourite ways of cooking vegetables, including recipes given to me by other keen vegetable cooks. Many of them are very simple ideas exploiting the natural adaptability of vegetables and enhancing their natural flavour. Others are more involved, but never tricksy – vegetables don't need grand artifice. There are salads, starters and side dishes, main courses, puddings and preserves. Some recipes include meat or fish, others are suitable for vegetarians and carnivores alike. Many of the dishes deserve to be served as a course on their own, so that they can be savoured without getting swamped on a plate piled high with other bits and bobs.

The problem with writing a book on vegetables is that there are just so many of them and so many ways to cook each one. Limited space has meant imposing my own limits on what is included. There are notable omissions – seakale, salsify, sweet potatoes, to name but a few – and many recipes that I would have liked to include but were squeezed out for lack of room. Maybe one day I'll get the opportunity to add a second volume . . . .

I hope that what is here will inspire readers to take a new look at vegetables and to explore their potential to the full. It would delight me to think that a few more children might grow up enjoying their greens and not being forced to eat them only because they are 'good for you'. Allowing vegetables to shine in all their diversity makes absolute sense. Sure, they are good for you. They are also cheap and abundant, but above all vegetables should be a pleasure to cook and an even greater pleasure to eat.

SOPHIE GRIGSON

Notes on Using the Recipes

Vegetables do not come in standard sizes, so in some instances you will have to use your own judgement as to, say, how large a large aubergine is, or how long it will take the pumpkin you've bought to cook. Where no specific size or weight is stated, assume that it means an average or medium-sized specimen. Cooking times are there as guidelines only, so don't rely absolutely on my 15 minutes or whatever. Check for yourself and allow a few less or a few extra minutes if necessary.

Always stick with either the metric measurements or the imperial ones, never a mixture of the two. Spoon measurements are rounded, unless otherwise stated. Eggs are size 2.

Taste as you cook wherever possible, and adjust flavourings to your liking. I happen to be particularly fond of garlic, chilli and fresh herbs. It's up to you to decide whether your taste for these ingredients matches mine. You may prefer your food less or more highly seasoned. When I use olive oil it is always extra virgin olive oil, a blended commercial brand for general cooking and a classier, more highly flavoured single-estate olive oil for salads and as a condiment at the end of cooking. Plain olive oil, what used to be known as 'pure olive oil' has a milder flavour and you may prefer that for general use. Wherever I think the stronger taste of extra virgin oil is essential, I've listed it specifically amongst the ingredients.

SHOOTS

Asparagus ● *Cardoons*
Globe Artichokes
Celery ● *Fennel*

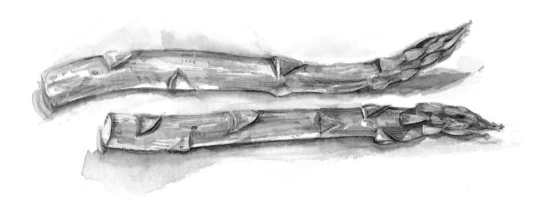

Asparagus

The Vale of Evesham has long been famous for its fine asparagus. It used to be grown on a grand scale in the village of Bretforton, though now the asparagus fields have dwindled to a few acres. Even so, the old traditions linger on and once a year on the last Sunday in May, the village pub holds a grand asparagus auction. The day before, market gardener Peter Tomkins is hard at work.

What marks out his asparagus from the rest is the way he ties it. Using ancient well-worn asparagus cradles on his old slotted bench, he deftly bends narrow strips of soft willow to secure prime purple-tipped asparagus in neat, tight blocks of one hundred or one 'half-hundred'. I've never seen asparagus look more beautiful. It is a dying art: when old-timers like Peter Tomkins have gone, we will have lost a skill that pays tribute to this most delicate and luxurious of vegetables.

I look forward eagerly to the beginning of the asparagus season when, like Peter Tomkins and his wife, I take the purist attitude that the only way to do justice to asparagus is to serve it plainly cooked, with melted butter, olive oil or Hollandaise sauce (see p. 17). (The Tomkins family are even more categorical: you must only boil asparagus with a little mint and eat it with butter and black pepper.) However, as the supply increases I turn to other recipes, determined to make the most of the season.

Green-stemmed asparagus, the type we grow in Britain, is graded into three sizes. The fashionable sprue is the spindly, extremely tender type which requires only a few minutes' cooking. Growers, however, consider sprue the poor relation – not much to sink your teeth into. 'Best' is medium-thick, around 1 cm (½ inch) in diameter. Then there are the Specials: big and fat and juicy, the prime asparagus fit for a king.

Whatever its girth asparagus, or 'grass' as it is known in growing circles, should be firm and smooth (no tired wrinkles) and sprightly green, with no slimy patches marring its beauty. The tips should be tightly packed. Tips that are opening up belong to elderly asparagus, picked past its best.

Preparing Asparagus

To prepare, trim off an inch or two of the woody base. If the lower part of the stem looks as if it might be tough, then it may be a good idea to peel it (if I'm serving the asparagus whole, to be eaten with the fingers, then I rarely bother to do this – it's no trouble to chew it down to the stringy part, and leave that, sucked clean, on the side of the plate). Always save any trimmings (and water used to cook the asparagus) to make soup, or vegetable stock. They can both be frozen if you don't have much time to spare straight away.

With tender asparagus I usually steam the whole stem and tip in a normal steamer, but the accepted wisdom is that asparagus should be part-boiled, part-steamed, standing upright, with the tougher parts of the stems immersed in water, while the tender tips cook in the heat of the steam. If you don't have a proper asparagus steamer, use the tallest pan you have, tie the asparagus in a bundle with string and secure it in an upright position with scrumpled balls of silver foil tucked around the base to keep it steady or better still, with halved new potatoes which will absorb some of the asparagus flavour as they cook.

Pour in enough water to come about 4−5 cm (1½−2 inches) up the stems of the asparagus, bring to the boil, then cover the pan with a dome of silver foil to trap the steam. Reduce the heat slightly and simmer until the bases are tender. Lift out carefully and drain. If you are serving asparagus cold, run under the cold tap as soon as the spears are tender to halt cooking, and then drain thoroughly.

This classic method is not the only way of cooking asparagus. It can be roasted in the oven (see p. 22) or grilled (see p. 17) if it is not too thick. Be bold – you'll be surprised at the results.

Asparagus with Smoked Salmon and Sauce Mousseline

Dunworley Cottage Restaurant in West Cork is hard to find, but worth getting lost for once or twice. Perched on a headland with its wonderful views of the sea, it is run by Swede Katherine Noren who, with her chef Mikka, creates the most delicious food. She uses the best Irish produce and prepares it with a Swedish accent – like local black and white puddings with a lingonberry sauce. Katherine grows her own vegetables and herbs, bakes her own delicious bread and pickles

OVERLEAF *Katherine Noren's Asparagus with Smoked Salmon and Sauce Mousseline*

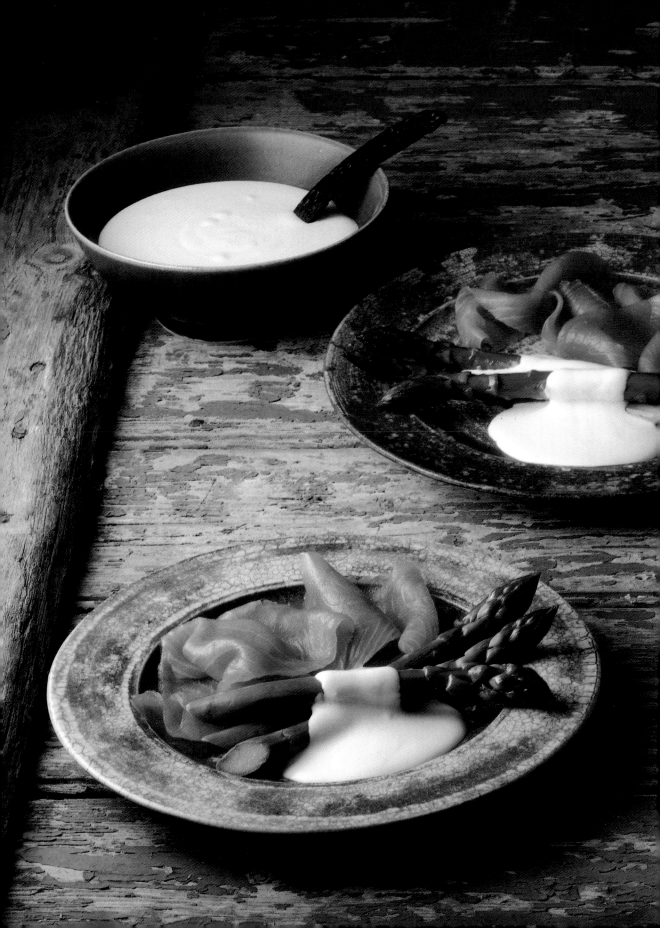

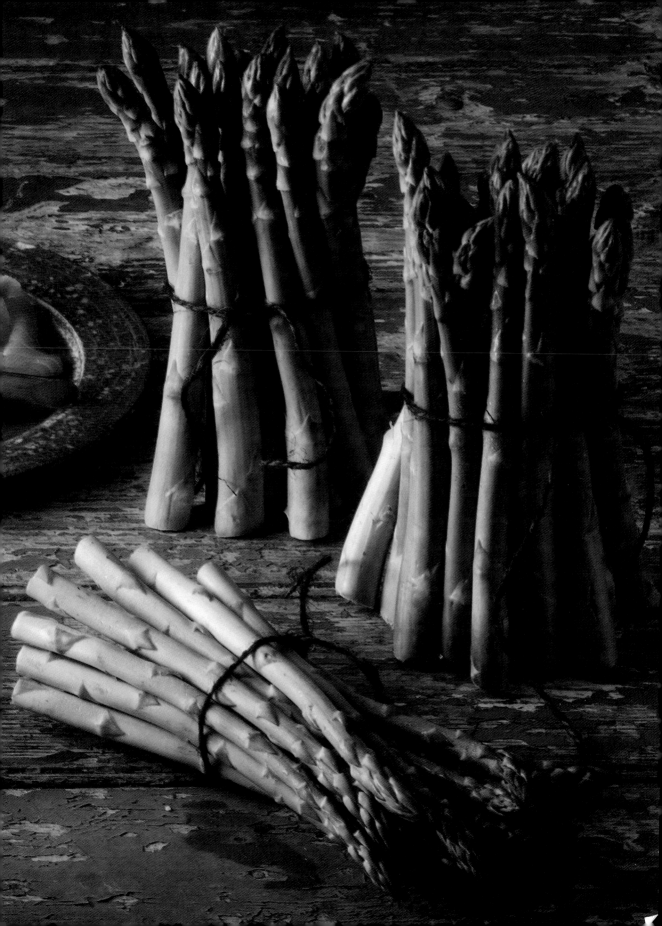

her own excellent herrings. She buys superb smoked salmon from a fish smoker a few miles down the coast and when asparagus is in season she serves them together with this luxuriously rich Sauce mousseline – Hollandaise (see opposite) sauce lightened with whipped cream.

SERVES 6

1 quantity of Hollandaise sauce (see opposite)
150 ml (5 fl oz) whipping cream, whipped

750 g (1½ lb) asparagus, trimmed, steamed and allowed to cool
6 slices smoked salmon
6 sprigs fresh parsley to garnish

Shortly before serving make the Hollandaise sauce, then fold in the whipped cream. Taste and adjust seasoning if necessary and keep warm. Arrange the cold, cooked asparagus and smoked salmon on 6 individual plates. Spoon a little of the sauce on to each plate and garnish with a sprig of parsley. Serve the remaining sauce in a bowl for those who really want to indulge themselves.

Asparagus and Sorrel Soup

A recipe to use up those precious asparagus trimmings. When preparing asparagus don't throw anything away. Save the trimmings (stringy stalk ends and parings) and cooking water which will be loaded with the flavour of fresh asparagus. Then you can make this simple but very delicious soup.

SERVES 2–3

175 g (6 oz) asparagus trimmings
40 g (1½ oz) butter
1 onion, chopped
1 clove garlic, peeled and chopped
1 handful of sorrel, shredded
1 tablespoon plain flour
600 ml (1 pint) water left from cooking asparagus *or* asparagus water and chicken stock

Salt and freshly ground black pepper
50 ml (2 fl oz) whipping *or* double cream (*optional*)
1 tablespoon fresh chervil *or* fresh chives, chopped

Chop the asparagus trimmings roughly. Melt the butter in a saucepan and cook the onion and garlic until tender, without browning. Add the shredded sorrel and stir until it collapses to a mush. Sprinkle the flour over, stir for a few seconds then, a little at a time, mix in the asparagus water and/or stock. Add the asparagus trimmings and salt and pepper. Simmer for 20 minutes.

Process or purée until smooth, then sieve to get rid of stringy fibres. Just before serving, re-heat to just under boiling point. Stir in the cream, if using, and chervil (or chives). Taste, adjust seasoning and serve.

Asparagus with Hollandaise Sauce

There's no finer way to celebrate the arrival of the asparagus season than by tucking into a plate of hot, steamed asparagus with a rich Hollandaise sauce. The classic method for making Hollandaise is not that difficult, but it can occasionally go wrong. I always play safe and make my Hollandaise in the food processor while the asparagus is cooking.

SERVES 6

1 kg (2 lb) asparagus

For the Hollandaise sauce
4 egg yolks
2 tablespoons lemon juice
1 tablespoon water
225 g (8 oz) unsalted butter, diced
Salt and freshly ground black pepper

Trim and steam the asparagus (see p. 13). While it is cooking, make the Hollandaise.

Put the egg yolks into the bowl of a food processor or liquidizer with a pinch of salt and whizz for a few seconds. Heat the lemon juice and water in a small saucepan until just boiling. At the same time, put the butter into another saucepan and heat gently until foaming.

Turn on the processor and trickle in the hot lemon and water, keeping the machine whirring until it is all incorporated. Turn off. As soon as the butter is foaming, turn the processor on again and start adding the butter drop by drop. Once about a third of the butter is incorporated accelerate the adding of the butter to a slow but continuous trickle. After two thirds of the butter has been incorporated you can increase the flow slightly more. Stop short of the white sediment lurking at the bottom of the pan. Taste and adjust seasoning, adding a little more lemon juice if needed. Serve immediately with the asparagus, or keep warm in a bowl over a pan of barely simmering water until required.

Grilled Spring Onions and Asparagus with Lime and Coarse Sea Salt

Grilling spring onions and asparagus gives them a smoky flavour that is enhanced by the spicy sharpness of lime. Serve a mixture of the two, or make it even simpler by using just asparagus or just spring onions. The asparagus should be fairly thin; not sprue but no more than 1 cm (½ inch) in diameter.

OVERLEAF *Grilled Spring Onions and Asparagus with Lime and Coarse Sea Salt*

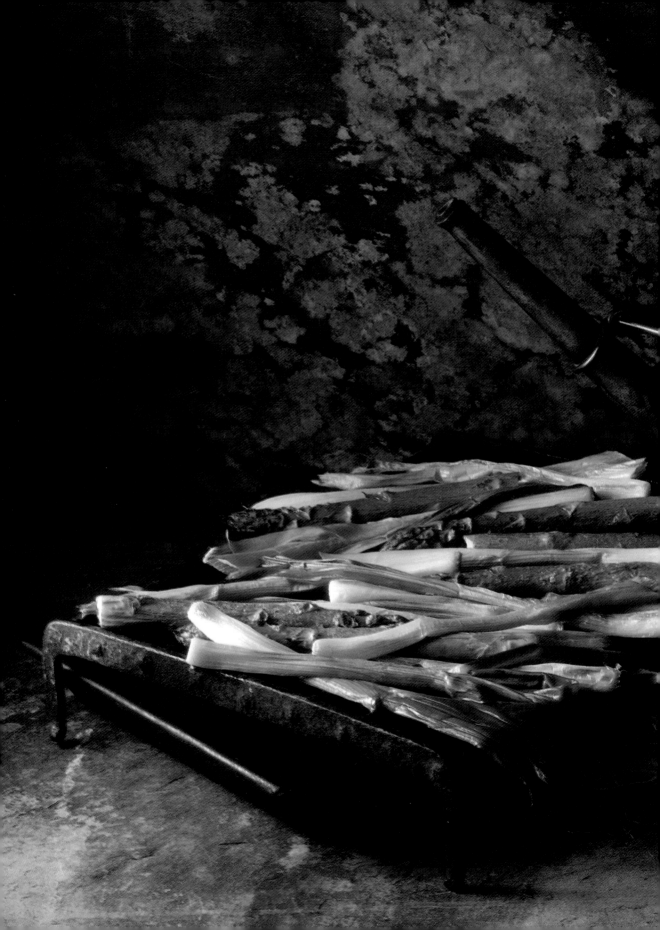

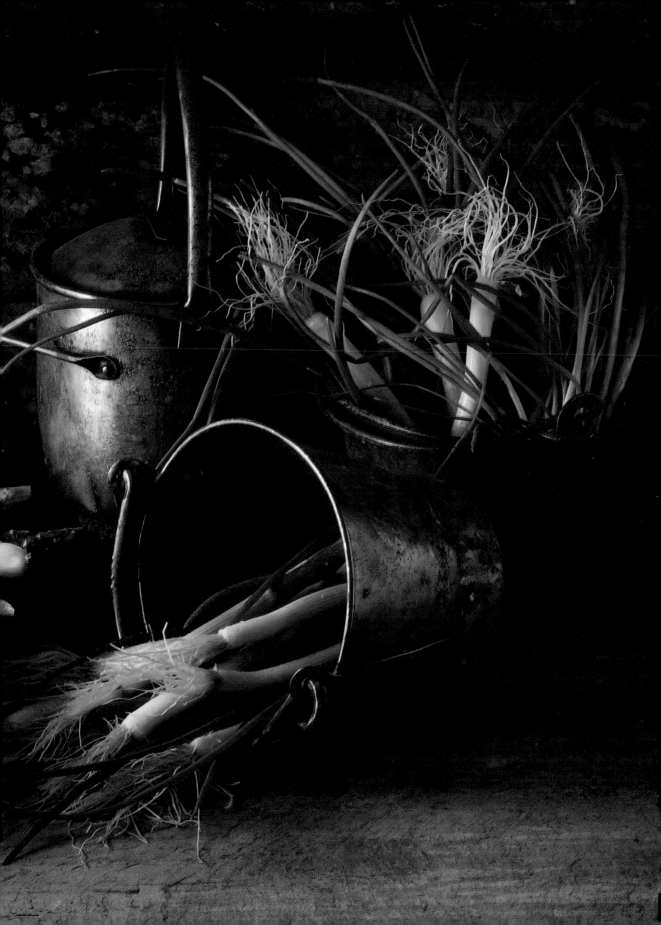

PER PERSON

4 fat spring onions *or* very thin baby
    leeks, trimmed

4 asparagus spears, trimmed

Olive *or* sunflower oil

Wedges of lime

Coarse sea salt

Brush the spring onions and asparagus with the oil and grill, turning until patched with brown. Serve immediately with lime and sea salt.

Asparagus and Gruyère Quiche

This is a quiche to make at the height of the asparagus season when you've feasted your fill of plainly cooked asparagus – a good way of stretching a small quantity of asparagus.

SERVES 6–8

For 350 g (12 oz) shortcrust pastry

225 g (8 oz) plain flour

Pinch of salt

100 g (4 oz) chilled butter, diced

1 egg yolk, beaten

Iced water

For the filling

350 g (12 oz) asparagus

100 g (4 oz) Gruyère cheese

3 shallots *or* 1 small onion, chopped

15 g (½ oz) butter

3 eggs

150 ml (5 fl oz) milk

85 ml (3 fl oz) double cream

1 tablespoon chopped fresh chervil
    or fresh parsley

Salt and freshly ground black pepper

First make the pastry. Sift the flour with the salt. Rub the butter into the flour until it resembles fine breadcrumbs. Make a well in the centre and add the egg yolk and enough iced water to form a soft dough – 1½–2 tablespoons of water should be enough. Mix quickly and lightly, and knead very briefly to smooth out. Wrap and chill for at least 30 minutes in the fridge. Bring back to room temperature before using.

Pre-heat the oven to gas mark 6, 400°F (200°C).

Line a 23-cm (9-inch) tart tin with the pastry. Leave it to rest in the fridge for 30 minutes. Prick the base with a fork and line with greaseproof paper or foil and weigh down with baking beans. Bake for 10 minutes. Remove paper or foil and beans and return to the oven for 5 minutes to dry out. Cool.

Trim the asparagus, breaking off the tough ends (save these and cooking water for making soup. Cut into 2-cm (¾-inch) lengths, keeping the tips separate. Pour 4 cm (1½ inches) of water into a large saucepan, add salt, and bring to the boil. Add the stem pieces and simmer for 5 minutes. Add tips and simmer gently for 2–3 minutes, until almost *al dente*, but still firm. Drain. If prepared in advance, cool and cover.

Dice 75 g (3 oz) of the Gruyère and grate the remaining 25 g (1 oz). Fry the shallots or onion gently in the butter until tender, without browning. Scatter asparagus, diced Gruyère and shallots over the base of the pastry case.

Whisk the eggs lightly, then whisk in the milk, cream, chervil or parsley and salt and pepper. Pour over the asparagus and Gruyère. Scatter remaining Gruyère over the top. Bake at gas mark 4, 350°F (180°C) for 25–30 minutes, until just set in the centre and nicely browned. Serve hot, warm or cold.

Pasta with Asparagus and Horseradish

A simple dish with lively flavours, that can be conjured up quickly. Horseradish may not sound like the ideal companion for delicate asparagus but used in moderation, as it is here, it marries surprisingly well. For a richer dish, add 150 ml (5 fl oz) of double cream to the asparagus when re-heating.

SERVES 4

450 g (1 lb) asparagus
Salt
450 g (1 lb) fusilli *or* other pasta shapes
50 g (2 oz) butter

1 tablespoon creamed horseradish
Squeeze of lemon juice
2 tablespoons chopped fresh chives to
    garnish

Trim the asparagus, breaking off the tough ends (save these and cooking water for making soup). Cut into 2-cm (¾-inch) lengths, keeping the tips separate. Pour 4 cm (1½ inches) of water into a large saucepan, add salt, and bring to the boil. Add the stem pieces and simmer for 5 minutes. Add tips and simmer gently for 3–4 minutes, until just tender. Drain. If prepared in advance, cool and cover.

Bring a large pan of salted water to a gentle, rolling boil, tip in the pasta and cook until *al dente*. A few minutes before the pasta is done, melt the butter in a frying-pan. Add the asparagus and stir to re-heat thoroughly, without actually frying. Add the horseradish and lemon juice and stir.

Drain the pasta well, and tip into a hot serving dish. Spoon the asparagus mixture over the pasta, toss, scatter with chopped chives and serve.

Asparagus and New Potatoes with Parmesan

Asparagus and new potatoes are perfect bedfellows, each benefiting from the other's presence. In this dish both can be cooked in advance, leaving only the final re-heating and browning to be done just before serving.

SERVES 4 as a first course or side dish

225 g (8 oz) asparagus
225 g (8 oz) new potatoes
3 tablespoons olive oil
2 cloves garlic, peeled and chopped

½–¾ teaspoon chilli flakes
25 g (1 oz) Parmesan, cut into paper-thin
    slivers

Trim the asparagus discarding the woody ends. Cut into 2.5-cm (1-inch) lengths, keeping tips and stalks separate. Bring a pan of lightly salted water to the boil. Add the stems and simmer for 5 minutes. Now add the tips and simmer for a further 3–4 minutes until tender. Drain and rinse under the cold tap. Drain and dry on kitchen paper.

Halve the potatoes or quarter if large. Steam or boil in the asparagus water, until just tender, topping up with extra water if necessary. Drain well and dry.

Turn on the grill so that it has time to heat up. Heat the oil in a wide frying-pan and add the garlic and chilli. Cook gently for 2–3 minutes. Raise the heat slightly and add the asparagus and potatoes. Toss in the oil for a few minutes to heat through. Tip into a shallow heatproof dish, scatter over the Parmesan and whisk under the grill. Grill until lightly patched with brown and serve.

Roast Asparagus with Parmesan

It was my friend and colleague, Henrietta Green, who introduced me to the joys of roast asparagus. Incredulous at first I'm now an out-and-out convert. It's by far the easiest way to cook asparagus for a dinner party, and the flavour of the stems is intense and undiminished.

Exact cooking time depends on the thickness of the asparagus. Smaller stems will take no more than 10 minutes, thicker ones up to 18 or so. Test with a skewer (a couple of inches from the base of the stem) to see if they are tender. Since it is the method rather than the quantities that count here, the recipe can easily be adapted to fit the amount of asparagus you have to hand.

SERVES 3–4

450 g (1 lb) asparagus　　　　　　　Freshly grated Parmesan to serve
6–8 tablespoons olive oil　　　　　　　(*optional*)
Coarse sea salt

Pre-heat the oven to gas mark 4, 350°F (180°C).

Cut the woody ends of stems off the asparagus and, if you think it necessary, peel the bottom couple of inches.

Generously oil a large ovenproof dish or roasting tin (big enough to take the asparagus in a tight single layer). Sprinkle coarse sea salt lightly over the base. Arrange the asparagus on top and drizzle over the remaining olive oil, erring on the generous side. Turn the asparagus with your hands to coat them nicely in oil. Sprinkle with a little more salt. Roast for 10–18 minutes until tender. Scatter with Parmesan if you wish, and serve immediately.

Cardoons

Coming face-to-face with a cardoon for the first time can be a daunting experience. These strange, stark, dramatic vegetables are no longer a familiar sight in Britain, though they grow here happily. Cardoons are a type of giant edible thistle, closely related to the globe artichoke, though it is the stems that are eaten rather than the flowering heads. The taste lies somewhere between celery and globe artichoke with a pleasing hint of bitterness.

Cardoons are a local favourite in parts of the Mediterranean. In the autumnal markets of the Piedmont region, you can see them piled so high that the stall-holder is all but hidden behind the mass of foliage. They are eaten in parts of Spain and Morocco, and in Provence too, but you are very unlikely to find fully grown cardoons for sale in this country. The only answer is to grow them yourself. If you are lucky your local gardening centre may stock small cardoon plants or packets of seeds. They grow easily so it's worth a try if you have the space in your garden.

If Clarissa Dickson Wright had her way, they would be a familiar sight on every dining-table in Britain – as they were before they fell out of favour with the Victorians. Clarissa runs Books for Cooks, the London shop specializing in books on food and wine. She is a woman with a mission – to reintroduce the cardoon to the British. She has borrowed a patch of land from a friend near Skegness, where she, with his help, grows a small forest of cardoons amongst the sea of caravans. Her collection of cardoon recipes is unparalleled, and you'll find two of them on the following pages.

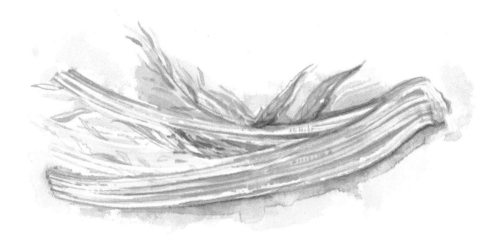

Preparing Cardoons

So how should you approach these intriguing looking vegetables, with their long, long stems fringed with a mass of silvery leaves? Sadly, the leaves are of no use and must be chopped off and discarded along with the sometimes spiky leaflets that run the length of the stems. With that heap of debris in the bin you can tackle the vegetable proper.

Very young stems may be tender and mild enough to eat raw, but nibble a small piece first. It's more likely that they will need to be blanched to remove excessive bitterness. Cut the stems into manageable lengths, pulling off tough strings as you do so. For most purposes 4–5 cm (1½–2 inches) lengths will be about right. Drop them into a pan of boiling water generously acidulated with lemon juice. Simmer for 10–15 minutes, drain, and have another test nibble. A mild hint of bitterness is no bad thing, but more than that and they should be simmered again in fresh water for another 5 minutes or so. Luckily the stems are quite robust and can take this kind of treatment without collapsing to a mush. Once they've been adequately blanched, drain thoroughly.

You can eat them more or less as they are, perhaps re-heated in butter, or tossed in a well-flavoured vinaigrette to make a salad. However, they benefit from the support of strong flavours, such as cheese, anchovies, olives, spices and garlic. They are the classic vegetable to serve with a bagna cauda (the Piedmontese anchovy and garlic dip, see p. 26), and they make an excellent gratin, bathed in a Parmesan sauce, or a tomato one, topped with breadcrumbs and cheese.

They also make good casings for stuffings – try the recipe cooked for me by Clarissa Dickson Wright (see below), or make up your own variation. Who knows, you may even become as passionate about them as the Cardoon Queen herself.

Clarissa Dickson Wright's
North African Jewish Cardoons

Cardoons are popular vegetables in parts of North Africa, and this favourite recipe of Clarissa Dickson Wright is one of the many ways they are used there. The wide, welcoming stems of cardoon make perfect containers for fillings, such as this spicy lamb stuffing. The trick is to fry the filled cardoon very slowly. Serve them with a fresh green vegetable or a green or tomato salad. We ate them outside Books for Cooks, which Clarissa runs, attracting the attention of a couple of French visitors, one of whom was a chef from Toulouse. Curiously he had never heard of cardoons though they are grown not so very far away from Toulouse, in Provence. However, they both loved them – and promptly polished off the lot!

SERVES 4

4–6 cardoon stalks	Flour for coating
Juce of ½ lemon	Salt and freshly ground black
2 eggs, lightly beaten	pepper
	Olive oil for frying

For the stuffing

225 g (8 oz) minced lamb	1 teaspoon ground cumin
2 cloves garlic, peeled and finely chopped	100 g (4 oz) par-cooked potato finely diced (*optional*)
1 onion, finely chopped	Salt and freshly ground black pepper
1 bunch fresh coriander, chopped	

Mix together all the stuffing ingredients, cover, and leave in a cool place for 1 hour.

Trim the cardoon stalks and cut into 5-cm (2-inch) lengths. Blanch for 10 minutes in water acidulated with the lemon juice, then drain and plunge into cold water. Drain again thoroughly.

Take golf-ball sized pieces of the stuffing, shape into short, stubby sausages and sandwich each one snugly between 2 pieces of cardoon, pressing together. Pour the eggs into a shallow bowl. Season the flour with salt and pepper and spread out on a plate.

Heat a generous depth of oil in a wide frying-pan over a medium to low heat. Coat the cardoon 'sandwiches' in the flour and *then* dip into the egg. Fry slowly for a good 15 minutes, turning occasionally, until they are browned. Don't rush the frying as the heat needs to penetrate through the cardoon to cook the stuffing. Drain and serve immediately.

Provençal Gratin of Cardoons

This gratin of cardoons is served on Christmas Eve in Provence as part of the 'fasting supper'. Far from being a mean little affair this is a grand feast to welcome in Christmas Day. 'Fasting' merely means that there is no meat. Clarissa Dickson Wright found the recipe in Elizabeth Luard's European Festival Food *(Bantam Press) and has since made a few small adjustments to suit her taste. The truffle is by no means mandatory, though for special occasions it adds a note of luxury.*

SERVES 4

4–6 inner stalks of cardoon	2 tablespoons plain flour
Juice of ½ lemon	300 ml (10 fl oz) white wine
4 tablespoons olive oil	4 tablespoons grated cheese (e.g. Gruyère
10 black olives, pitted and roughly chopped	*or* Emmenthal)
1 black truffle (*optional*), fresh or bottled and very thinly sliced	Salt and freshly ground black pepper

Trim the cardoons and cut into 2.5–5 cm (1–2 inch) lengths. Blanch for 10–15 mintues in water acidulated with the lemon juice. Drain thoroughly.

Heat the olive oil in a large frying-pan. Add the cardoons and fry gently for 5 minutes. Add the olives and the truffle, if using. Stir for 1 minute or so. Sprinkle the flour over and stir to mix evenly. Stir in the wine and simmer for 10–15 minutes, stirring occasionally and adding a little more wine or a splash of water if it threatens to catch. The aim is to coat the cardoons in just a little thick sauce – they shouldn't be swimming in it. Season and spoon into an ovenproof gratin dish. Scatter over the grated cheese and place under a hot grill until browned and bubbling. Serve immediately.

Cardoons with Bagna Cauda

Bagna cauda is a pungent anchovy and garlic sauce or dip from the Piedmont. Out of season and out of its home district, it is usually served with a mixture of crudités and lightly blanched vegetables. However, the proper vegetable to dip into it is undoubtedly the cardoon. Bagna cauda is sometimes softened by the addition of a little cream, but I prefer the plainer version. By the way, if you use 200 ml (7 fl oz) of olive oil and leave out the butter, it also makes a blissful dressing for a grilled pepper salad.

SERVES 4–6
For the Bagna cauda
1 tin of anchovies, with the oil
150 ml (5 fl oz) olive oil
4 large cloves garlic, peeled and finely
    chopped
74 g (3 oz) butter
Freshly ground black pepper

To serve
Pieces of cooked cardoon (see p. 24)
Strips of raw vegetables: fennel, peppers
    (these can also be grilled), celery,
    carrot, etc.
Good bread

To make the Bagna cauda first chop the anchovies roughly. Put the oil from the tin and the olive oil into a saucepan and warm over a low heat. Add the chopped anchovies and garlic and cook gently, mashing down the anchovies with a fork, until they have dissolved and the garlic is beginning to colour and soften. Stir in the butter and season generously with pepper.

Arrange the vegetables on a serving plate. The Bagna cauda should be served hot so if you have a fondue set pour it into the pan and light the flame underneath. Otherwise pour it into a warmed bowl. Serve alongside the vegetables and encourage guests to stir up the Bagna cauda as they dip, so that they get some of the delicous anchovy and garlic cream that inevitably settles at the bottom.

Globe Artichokes

The last thing you expect to see at the end of the wild Beara Peninsula on the west coast of Ireland is a field of lovingly tended globe artichokes. But if you take a tiny, twisting turning off the Allihies road you will eventually come to Tony Lowes' ramshackle farmhouse, and what must surely be the most beautifully positioned fields of globe artichokes in the world: rows and rows of silvery-green vegetables, set against the backdrop of the Atlantic ocean. People come from miles around to buy globe artichokes from this American farmer who moved to Ireland in 1967 – partly because of their excellence, and partly because globe artichokes are something of a novelty in Ireland.

You can't rush globe artichokes. They are not designed to slot into a hectic schedule, in terms of growing, preparation, cooking, or eating. But they are, without doubt, worth making time for.

Globe artichokes vary in shape and size, according to variety, from squat, tightly packed balls to looser-leaved tapering ones. Choose them carefully, discarding any that seem dry and elderly. The leaves and stalk should be fleshy with no tell-tale brown patches.

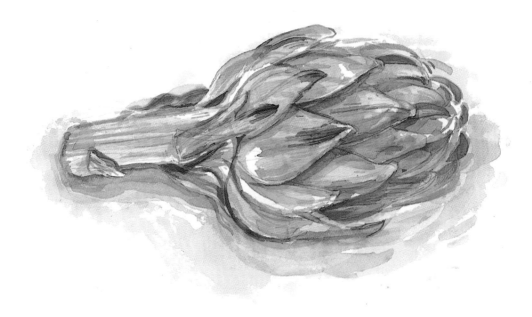

Preparing Globe Artichokes

Once selected, artichokes should be cooked as soon as possible. Unless you have a wealth of heads and can afford to use only the bases, cook and serve them whole. First get rid of any insects that have made their homes between the leaves by soaking them stem up in a bowl of well-salted water (wedge them together so that they don't bob upright) for 30 minutes or so. Then snap off the stem close to the base, pulling away the tougher fibres, and rub the exposed surface with lemon juice to prevent browning.

Cook in boiling, salted water, acidulated with the juice of half a lemon, or 2 tablespoons of vinegar, to every litre (2 pints) of water for 30–50 minutes depending on size, again wedging them to keep them upright, but this time with the stem end down. They are done as soon as an outer leaf can be pulled off easily bringing with it a tender scraping of base to chew off. Drain the artichokes well and eat hot or leave to cool.

If you only have one or two artichokes to cook they can be microwaved, each one wrapped tightly in clingfilm and cooked on full power for about 7 minutes for a singleton, 9–12 minutes for a brace, depending on the size of the artichoke and the power of the oven.

Blessed with a surfeit of artichokes, you can feel justified in discarding all the leaves in order to cook with the bases only (sometimes called the hearts, or bottoms). Use a sharp knife and have a halved lemon standing by. Snap off the stalk, pare the leaves off, working steadily round and round until all the tough ones have tumbled away, leaving just the tender cone. Ease off the cone, then use a small sharp knife to cut away the choke. Rub the cut surfaces with the lemon half as you work, to prevent browning, and drop the naked bases into a bowl of acidulated water as soon as possible.

A final thought: don't waste your best wine on globe artichokes, as they contain a chemical called cynarin which is soluble in water and lingers on in the saliva, its sweet taste destroying the flavour of the wine. Go for water instead, or even iced, neat vodka!

Barbecued Artichokes

Well, why not barbecue or grill globe artichokes? No good reason at all. They make a fine, if unusual, addition to a barbecued meal, served either as a first course or alongside the main dish. They do need to be prepared and partially cooked in advance, but with that out of the way the rest is plain sailing.

Preparing Artichoke Cups

For really classy presentation, turn the artichokes into cups which can hold their sauce or dressing in the centre. If they are to be served cold, prepare as usual: slice off the top inch or so of the leaves with a sharp knife, then boil or microwave. When cool enough to handle, gently ease open the leaves, exposing the tight, purplish cone of thin leaves in the centre. Twist this out to expose the hairy choke, which can then be scraped away with a teaspoon, leaving a well to be filled with whatever seems appropriate.

It's tougher work if you want to serve hot artichoke cups, since you'll need to work the raw artichokes before they are cooked. Prepare and slice off the tops. Open out the leaves, including the inner cone and using a tough teaspoon and a small sharp knife, scrape away the inner choke which, be warned, will cling stubbornly. With that done, you can now cook them in the ordinary way.

SERVES 4
2 large globe artichokes
Lemon juice
5 tablespoons olive oil
Salt and freshly ground black pepper

Snap off the stems of the artichokes close to the base. Rub the cut with lemon juice. Either boil the artichokes in water acidulated with the juice of ½ lemon for 10 minutes, or wrap individually in clingfilm, and microwave together on high for 3 minutes.

When they are cool enough to handle, trim off the outer ring of leaves (these can be tough). Quarter the artichokes. Rub all the cut edges with lemon juice as you work. Using a small sharp knife, scrape out the hairy choke. Cut each quarter in half.

Once you've done all the preparation, place the artichoke pieces in a single layer in a shallow dish. Whisk 2 tablespoons of lemon juice with the olive oil, salt and pepper. Pour this over the artichokes, making sure they are well coated. Cover, and keep cool until needed.

To cook, place over a hot barbecue, or under a pre-heated grill, one of the straight cut sides towards the heat. Grill for about 5–8 minutes until well patched with brown (don't worry about the leaves charring), then turn onto the second straight cut side, and cook for a further 5–8 minutes. By now they should be just tender – if necessary continue cooking, turning, for a few more minutes. Serve immediately.

OVERLEAF *Barbecued Artichokes*

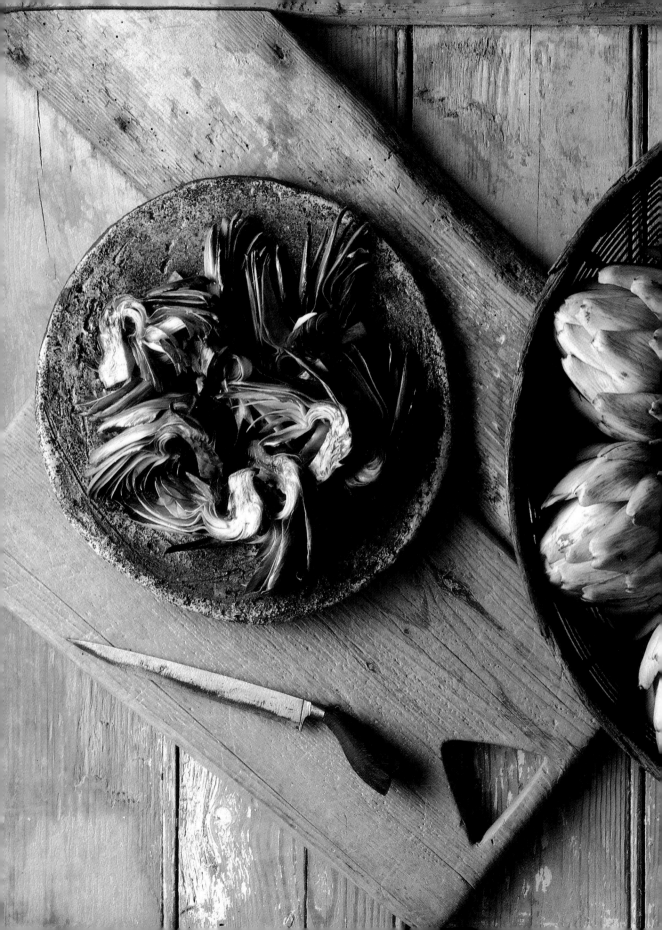

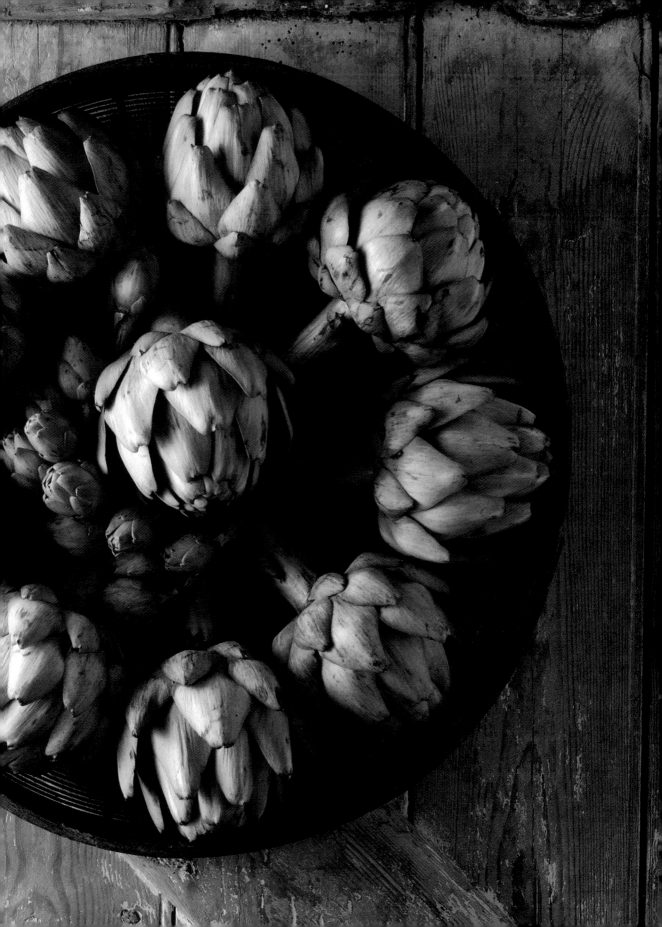

Eating Globe Artichokes

Eating globe artichokes is one of those delightful rituals of the table which leaves no room for great finesse. Fingers must be employed, at least until you reach the treasure of the base. Prepare thoroughly – lots of napkins, finger bowls if you are making a bid for smartness, and one (or more) large bowls in the centre of the table to take the debris.

When eating whole artichokes, complete with choke, put a large bowl or jug of the sauce or dressing on the table: with hot artichokes, melted butter sharpened with lemon juice or a rich Hollandaise (see p. 17), with cold ones, a vinaigrette, perhaps with finely chopped shallots in it, or crème fraîche beaten with lemon juice, herbs, salt, pepper and a pinch or two of sugar. Always prepare more than you think you'll need; with all the leaf dipping to follow it will disappear quickly.

Now the fun can begin. The first thing for each diner to do is to help themselves to sauce, spooning it onto the plate. To prevent it spreading out and under the artichoke first prop the far side of the plate up on the back of your fork (you don't need it for the moment), so that the plate slopes down towards you. The artichoke takes pride of place at the top of the slope, the sauce forms a fine dipping pool at the foot.

Working from the outside inwards, pull leaves off one at a time, dip the base into the sauce and nibble off the nugget of soft artichoke at the base. Stop when you hit the supple inner cone, grasp it firmly and twist off. Nibble off the artichoke around the base of the cone. Finally, tackle the artichoke bottom; pull or scrape off the choke in tufts and discard. Reclaim your fork, letting the plate settle back in its normal position. Eat the best bit, the sweet nutty base, spearing chunks of it and mopping up the sauce that remains on the plate.

Artichoke cups (see p. 29) require a slightly different technique. The sauce is all there, ready and waiting inside the artichoke, but in order to prevent it seeping out at quite the wrong moment, you must start with the upper leaves, gradually working your way outwards.

Globe Artichokes Filled with
Lemon Scrambled Eggs

Globe artichoke cups filled with lemony scrambled eggs make an elegant and substantial first course. Convenient too, as both artichokes and eggs can be prepared several hours in advance.

SERVES 4

4 globe artichokes	Salt and freshly ground black pepper
6 eggs	15 g (½ oz) butter
2 tablespoons lemon juice	2 tablespoons double cream
Finely grated zest of ½ lemon	1 tablespoon chopped fresh dill

To make the artichoke cups prepare as on p. 29, slicing off the top inch or so of the leaves with a sharp knife. Cook as on p. 28. When cool enough to handle, gently ease open the leaves, exposing the tight, purplish cone of thin leaves in the centre. Twist this out to expose the hairy choke, which can then be scraped away with a teaspoon, leaving a well to be filled with the scrambled egg mixture. Leave to cool completely.

Beat the eggs in a bowl with the lemon juice and zest, salt and pepper. Set the bowl over a pan of simmering water and add the butter and cream. Stir until the eggs are creamy (but not setting into hard lumps). Draw off the heat and stir in the dill. Cool slightly, then spoon into the artichoke cups. Serve cold.

Sautéed Artichokes, Potatoes and Carrots

Sautéed artichokes are quite irresistible and I would eat them by the plateful, if only some kind person would do all the preparation for me. Having no kitchen slave I compromise by sautéeing a couple of artichokes along with potatoes and carrots, and an excellent compromise it is too. If you are more patient than I am you can increase the quantity of artichokes. If you have no patience or no artichokes, then sautéed potatoes and carrots alone are almost as good.

SERVES 3–4

2 large globe artichokes	½ tablespoon finely chopped fresh parsley
Lemon juice	
350 g (12 oz) waxy salad potatoes	½ tablespoon chopped fresh fennel *or* fresh dill
3 tablespoons olive oil	
225 g (8 oz) medium carrots, sliced about 1 cm (½ inch) thick	½ tablespoon finely chopped fresh chives
	Salt and freshly ground black pepper

Snap the stems off the artichokes. Using a sharp knife, cut off the leaves and scrape off the choke. Turn in lemon juice as you work to prevent browning. Dice the naked bases into 1-cm (½-inch) cubes. Toss in lemon juice and pat dry. Peel and dice the potatoes into 1-cm (½-inch) cubes.

Heat the olive oil in a wide, heavy frying-pan. Add the potatoes, artichokes and carrots and sauté gently for about 15 minutes, turning frequently, until tender and browned. Drain briefly on kitchen paper, then toss with the herbs, salt and pepper. Serve immediately.

Sauce Rougette

In Brittany where a huge quantity of top-grade artichokes are grown, the locals serve them with this shallot vinaigrette.

SERVES 4

1½ tablespoons red wine vinegar
Salt and freshly ground black pepper
8 tablespoons groundnut *or* olive oil
3 shallots, finely chopped

Mix the vinegar with salt and pepper and whisk in the olive oil a little at a time. Add the shallots and serve.

Rabbit, Artichoke and New Potato Stew

This is so good that it is worth spending time preparing all those artichoke bases. Use up to eight, depending on size, availability or price, but don't be tempted to substitute canned artichoke bases – not at all the same thing. The rest is pretty simple and the result is superb.

SERVES 4

4–8 globe artichokes
Lemon juice
25 g (1 oz) butter
Plain flour for dusting
Salt and freshly ground black pepper
1 young rabbit, cut into joints

1 small onion, finely chopped
150 ml (5 fl oz) dry white wine
450 g (1 lb) small new potatoes
2 tablespoons finely chopped fresh
   parsley
A few leaves of fresh basil, torn up

Prepare the artichoke bases (see page 28) quarter and drop them into a bowl of water acidulated with a little lemon juice to prevent browning.

Heat the butter in a wide, heavy saucepan or oven-proof casserole dish, season the flour with salt and pepper and dust the rabbit pieces with it, and then brown them in the butter. Remove from pan and replace with the onion. Turn the heat down a little and cook until tender, without browning. Pour in the wine and bring to the boil, scraping in all the residues on the bottom of the pan.

Return the rabbit to the pan and season with salt and pepper. Cover and simmer for 15 minutes, then add potatoes, drained artichoke hearts and 1 tablespoon of parsley. Cover tightly and cook gently, stirring occasionally, for about 40 minutes until rabbit and vegetables are tender. Taste and adjust seasoning, sprinkle with remaining parsley and basil, and serve.

Celery

Celery is one of those love-it-or-loathe-it vegetables. There was a girl at my primary school who loathed even the smell of celery and we, pitiless children that we were, would chase her round the playground brandishing stems of celery whenever opportunity allowed. I love it on the other hand. I love its crispness and snap, and its flavour. Excellent served full length with real farmhouse British cheese, piled high with cream cheese, or chopped in salads.

Celery's potential as a cooked vegetable is all too often ignored, except perhaps as a flavouring for stocks. Boiled in water, it can be pretty tedious, I'll admit, but braised in the minimum of stock and served with a generous knob of butter it begins to take on an altogether more appealing aspect.

Frying is another option, and one of the best – check out the recipes that follow for two examples which I cooked with Mark Smith at Channings Wood Prison, one of the few prisons to run a professional catering course. Mark is an extremely funny, intelligent young Welshman who aims to run his own Welsh restaurant one day. Had it not been for the high walls and the fact that the kitchen knives were carefully counted and locked up at night, we could have been in an open university. The atmosphere was so cordial and the prisoners in their chef's whites and red neckerchiefs enjoyed their cooking so heartily. Mark made a deliciously simple, lightly curried, celery dish from a recipe by John Tovey, which I think is one of the nicest possible ways to enjoy cooked celery (see p. 37).

When it comes to buying celery, it always seems startlingly obvious to me that it should be fresh and firm, though all too often I've seen it for sale in a state of depressed limpness, stems patched with brown, and the fine head of leaves shorn off as if it were of no interest. The leaves have a powerful but delicious flavour, and can be used as a herb in soups or sauces, or chopped fresh into salads or cream cheese.

Preparing Celery

To prepare celery for the table separate the stalks and trim off dry ends. Pull off any strings down the outside. Stand in a jug of iced water, or place in a plastic bag with a sprinkling of water, knot and keep in the vegetable drawer of the fridge. Eat it soon, while it is still at its perky best.

For braising you have a choice – hearts or chopped. Hearts, i.e. the lower 10 cm (4 inches) or so of the whole clump, with the tips and outer stems removed, should be halved or quartered lengthways before braising. Even so, I find that you have to use so much stock just to cover them that they lose an enormous amount of flavour by the time they are cooked. I prefer to chop the celery into smaller pieces, 1–2.5 cm (½–1 inch) long removing strings as I do so. That way it can be packed tightly into the pan and requires only the minimum of liquid to keep it moist.

Guinea Fowl with Celery and Dill

Based on various French recipes, this casserole brings together guinea fowl and celery in a rich sauce – a perfect dish for a family Sunday lunch. If you can't get guinea fowl, it can be made with chicken or pheasant.

SERVES 4

1 plump guinea fowl
30 g (1 oz) butter
1 tablespoon sunflower oil
1 onion, chopped
2 cloves garlic, peeled and chopped
3 sprigs of fresh dill *or* ½ tablespoon dried
Bouquet garni
(2 sprigs thyme, 1 bay leaf, 3 sprigs parsley, tied together with string)

150 ml (5 fl oz) dry white wine
Salt and freshly ground black pepper
1 head of celery, sliced
15 g (½ oz) plain flour
150 ml (5 fl oz) double cream
Squeeze of lemon juice
1 tablespoon chopped fresh dill to garnish

Brown the guinea fowl briskly in 15 g (½ oz) butter and the oil and set aside. Fry the onion and garlic gently in the same fat without browning. Make a bed of the onion and garlic in a flameproof casserole just large enough to take the guinea fowl and, eventually, the celery. Add the dill. Set the guinea fowl on top, breast-side down. Tuck the bouquet garni in alongside and pour over the wine and 150 ml (5 fl oz) of water. Season with salt and pepper. Bring to a simmer, then reduce heat and cover tightly. Simmer lazily for 30 minutes. Turn the bird the right way up and snuggle the celery tightly around it. Cover tightly again, and continue cooking for a further 40 minutes until both guinea fowl and celery are tender. Place the bird on a serving dish, scoop out celery with a slotted spoon and place around it. Keep warm. Discard bouquet garni and bedraggled sprigs of dill.

Make beurre manié by mashing the remaining 15 g (½ oz) of butter thoroughly with the flour. Stir small knobs of it into the cooking juices left in the casserole, and cook at just under a simmer for 4 minutes. Stir in the cream, bring back to a simmer, then stir in a squeeze of lemon juice. Taste and adjust seasoning. Pour a little of the sauce over the celery, sprinkle with chopped dill. Serve the remaining sauce separately.

Stir-fried Celery with Ginger and Coriander

This is a lively, fresh-tasting way of cooking celery with ginger, coriander and orange juice.

SERVES 4

2 tablespoons vegetable *or* sunflower oil	1 teaspoon coriander seeds, coarsely crushed
2.5-cm (1-inch) piece of fresh ginger, peeled and finely chopped	Juice of ½ large orange
6 stalks celery, thinly sliced	Salt and freshly ground black pepper
	1 tablespoon chopped fresh coriander

Heat the oil in a large wok over a high heat. Add the ginger and stir for a few seconds. Now add the celery and stir-fry for about 2 minutes. Add the crushed coriander seeds and continue to stir-fry for about another 3 minutes until the celery is browned. Reduce heat, add the orange juice, salt and pepper. Toss, then cover and simmer for 4 minutes or so, until the liquid is absorbed. Stir in the chopped coriander and serve.

John Tovey's Lightly Curried, Deep-fried Celery Strips

Mark Smith is one of the keenest students on the Channings Wood Prison's professional catering course. He loves food and loves cooking. When I visited the kitchens he conjured up this remarkably delicious and simple dish of deep-fried celery strips. The other prisoners on the course and I gobbled them up so fast that he had to make a second batch straight away.

The deep-fried celery could be served with drinks before a meal, but would also go particularly well with roast game.

OVERLEAF *Guinea Fowl with Celery and Dill*

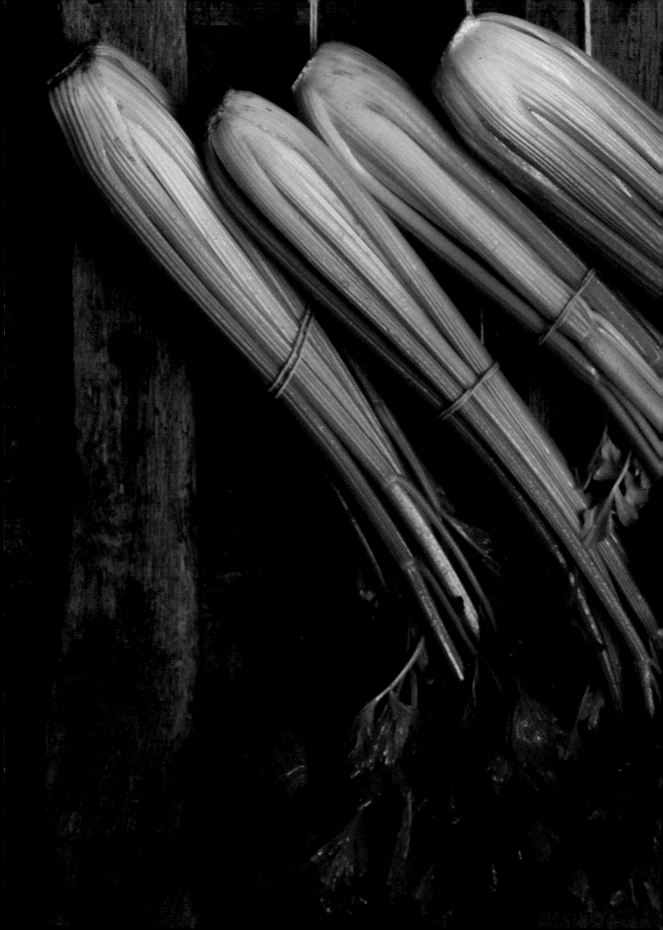

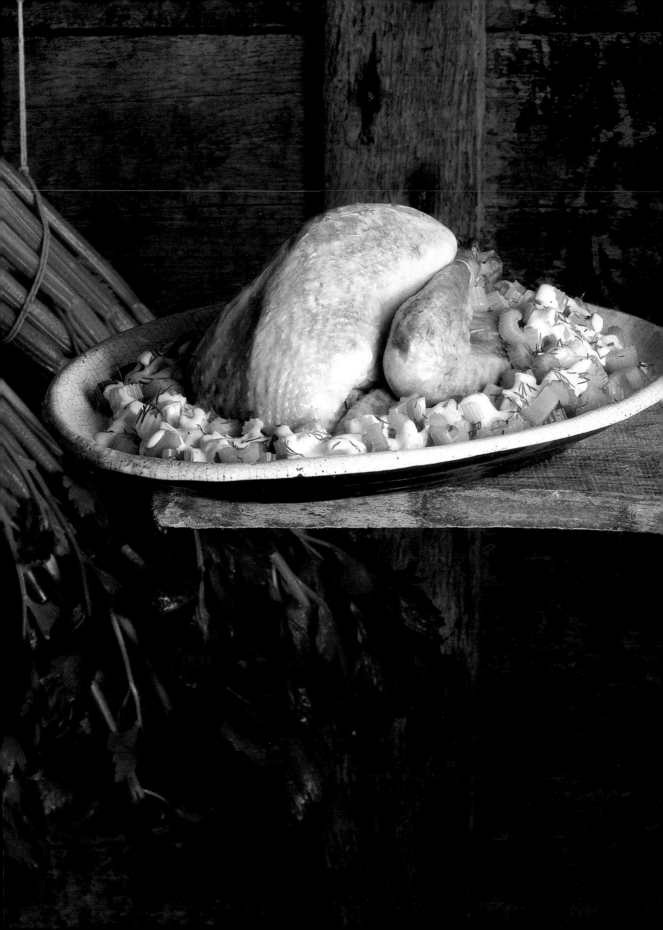

Serves 6

400–450 g (14–16 oz) celery stalks	5 teaspoons curry powder
Milk for soaking	Oil for deep-frying
75 g (3 oz) plain flour	Salt

Cut each stalk into 5-cm (2-inch) pieces and then into 5-mm (¼-inch) thick strips. Soak in cold milk until you want to fry them. Mix the flour and curry powder and spread out on a baking tray or put into a roomy plastic bag. Drain the celery strips in a sieve, then tip into the flour mixture, mixing to coat evenly. Tip back into the sieve to shake off excess flour.

Pre-heat a pan of oil to 360°F/182°C. Fry the strips in the oil for about 4 minutes in 3–4 batches, using the handle of a wooden spoon to stop them clogging together. Drain briefly on kitchen paper and serve immediately, sprinkled with salt.

Celery in Sweet and Sour Tomato Sauce

In this recipe, which I cooked at Channings Wood Prison, the celery is again fried – a treatment it takes to well – but this time in a shallow pan. The fried celery is mixed into a sweet and sour Sicilian-style tomato sauce, to be served cold as an hors d'œuvre or a vegetable side dish that is almost a relish.

Serves 4–6

1 head of celery or about 450 g (1 lb) celery stalks	2 tablespoons caster sugar
5 tablespoons olive oil	4 cloves
1 onion, chopped	1 cinnamon stick
1 × 400 g (14 oz) tin chopped tomatoes, or 450 g (1 lb) tomatoes, skinned and chopped	½ star anise, broken into 'petals' (*optional*)
	Salt and freshly ground black pepper
3 tablespoons sherry vinegar *or* red wine vinegar	14 black olives, pitted and sliced
	2 tablespoons chopped fresh parsley

Split the wider lower ends of the celery stalks in two, then slice the whole lot thinly. Use either two frying-pans to cook the celery, or cook in two batches. In each pan, heat 2½ tablespoons of oil and add half of the celery. Sauté over a brisk heat until browned – this takes quite some time as there's a good deal of water in celery to be evaporated off. Scoop out the celery.

Sauté the onion in the same oil in one of the pans, adding a little extra oil if necessary, until lightly browned. Add the tomatoes. Cook over a high heat for a few minutes until thick, then add the vinegar, sugar, cloves, cinnamon, star anise, if using, and a little salt and pepper. Return the celery to the pan. Simmer gently for a further 10 minutes. Stir in the olives and parsley. Taste and adjust the seasoning, then spoon into a serving dish and leave to cool.

Salade Cauchoise

This salad from the Pays de Caux in northern France sets the crispness of celery against the softness of potatoes, with strips of ham in a creamy dressing. I sometimes replace the crème fraîche with fromage frais – not authentic but still French and still good.

SERVES 6
750 g (1½ lb) waxy salad potatoes
    or new potatoes
6 stalks celery
100 g (4 oz) cooked ham
A few sprigs of fresh chervil *or* fresh
    parsley

For the dressing
4 teaspoons cider vinegar
1½ tablespoons chopped fresh chervil
    or fresh parsley
1½ tablespoons chopped fresh chives
Salt and freshly ground black pepper
8 tablespoons crème fraîche
    or fromage frais

To make the dressing stir the vinegar, herbs, salt and pepper into the crème fraîche or fromage frais. Taste and adjust seasoning. Scrub the potatoes and steam until tender. While still warm, cut into cubes and toss in half the dressing. Leave to cool. I think it is a waste of time to try to remove odd pieces of skin, but if you are feeling pernickety strip them off before cutting up the cooked potatoes.

Slice the celery, and cut the ham into strips. Mix with the potatoes and enough extra dressing to coat without overwhelming. Spoon into a serving dish and arrange sprigs of chervil or parsley on top.

Celery with Chestnuts

Celery and chestnuts have a natural affinity. I'd rather have this combination than brussel sprouts and chestnuts any day. Peeling the chestnuts is a bore, but a fairly brief one – don't be tempted to settle for canned chestnuts which are a poor substitute.

SERVES 4
15 chestnuts
Chicken, duck, beef *or* vegetable stock
1 small head of celery, sliced
Bouquet garni (see p. 36)
40 g (1½ oz) butter
Salt and freshly ground black pepper

With a sharp knife score a deep 'x' through the tough skin of each chestnut. Put them in a saucepan with enough water to cover generously. Bring to the boil and simmer for 2 minutes. One or two at a time, take the chestnuts out of the saucepan and peel off outer and inner skin. Discard any chestnuts that are discoloured. Rinse out the pan and return the chestnuts to it with enough fresh water or stock to cover. Simmer until tender, then drain and break into large pieces.

Place the celery in a pan in just enough stock to cover add the bouquet garni and simmer until barely tender. Drain, and discard the bouquet garni. Rinse the saucepan and return the celery to it with the chestnuts, butter, salt and pepper. Stir over a moderate heat for a few minutes until chestnuts and celery are thoroughly heated through and impregnated with butter. Serve.

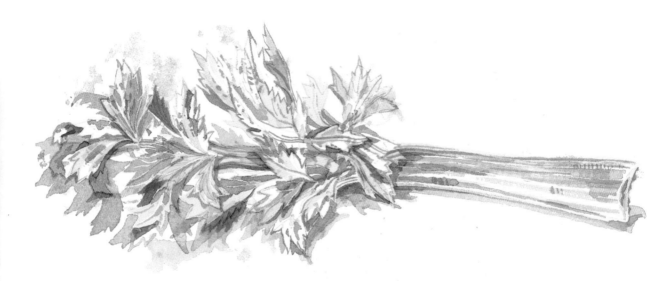

Fennel

Florence fennel is a marvellous vegetable with a unique aniseed taste. Or at least, I think it a marvellous vegetable, but I can understand why some people may dislike it. It announces its presence in no uncertain way, particularly when eaten raw. That's what I like about it. No namby-pamby background recluse, Florence fennel tastes strong and refreshing in a salad. Heat, though, induces a remarkable change, tempering the assertive flavour down to a mellow but distinctive sweetness when cooked.

Florence fennel and fennel herb are obviously closely related, but they are not identical plants. Florence fennel is grown for its tightly packed 'heads' or 'bulbs' which are actually the swollen basal stems of the plant. Having said that, the feathery leaves of Florence fennel can also be used as a herb.

How you use fennel will depend on how much you like it. It's not cheap to buy so choose your fennel carefully to minimize waste, and remind yourself that a little stretches a long way. Size is of no great importance: big fat bulbs are usually just as juicy and tender as more slender ones. The condition of the vegetable is what counts here. Look for firm, white orbs, with no soft or browning patches. The tufts of feathery green fronds should still be bright and fresh. If the fennel is in good condition when it enters your kitchen, it will keep for up to four days (or even a little longer)

Butter-fried Fennel and Onions with Vinegar and Thyme

Both my cousin, Lucy, and my aunt, Mary, are wonderful cooks, and I owe this dish entirely to them. Lucy came across the original recipe, which included no fennel at all, in The Green's Cook Book *by Deborah Madison (Bantam Press) which is one of the most inspiring of vegetarian cookery books. She and her mother adapted it between them, introducing the fennel. The whole ensemble doesn't take long to cook, but once done can be kept warm in the oven, covered, for up to 20 minutes or so.*

SERVES 4

1 large *or* 2 small fennel bulbs
2 medium red onions
50 g (2 oz) butter
2½ tablespoons sherry vinegar *or* red
    wine vinegar

Leaves of 3 sprigs of fresh thyme,
    roughly chopped
Salt and freshly ground black pepper

Preparing Fennel

To prepare fennel, trim a thin slice off the base and discard the stalks, which tend to be stringy. Use them to flavour stocks or sauces. Save the leaves, either to garnish the dish you are making, or to use as a herb with fish or chicken. If the outer layer of the fennel is looking ropy remove that as well.

When using fennel raw, either slice it thinly, or dice it small. It is excellent added to a tomato or cucumber salad, or in a mixed green salad. To cook it, halve or quarter the bulbs from top to base, depending on size, and simmer in salted water until just tender. Drain well and serve with a knob of butter, or re-heat in butter and oil, turning until lightly patched with brown. Thin slices can also be sautéed on their own to serve with grilled fish. Finely diced raw fennel, fried gently with onions and garlic, makes a delicious addition to a stuffing for poultry. Quartered bulbs of fennel can be grilled if brushed with oil first. But keep the heat gentle so that it penetrates through to the centre by the time the outside is browned. Fennel and potato soup is a favourite of mine too, slightly sharpened with a squeeze of lemon juice.

Trim the stalks off the fennel, halve lengthwise, and cut into slices 5 mm (¼ inch) thick, erring on the thin side. Halve the onions and cut into 5-mm (¼-inch) slices.

Melt the butter in a wide, heavy frying-pan. Add the fennel and cook gently for 5 minutes. Raise the heat to high, add the onions and sauté briskly, flipping and stirring them frequently. After 4–5 minutes they will be lightly browned, sweet and still a little crunchy. If you prefer them softer, cook for a couple of minutes longer. Now add the vinegar and sizzle until it is virtually all evaporated. Stir in the thyme leaves, salt and pepper and serve.

Dunworley Cottage Fennel Purée

I was given this recipe by Katherine Noren who runs the excellent Dunworley Cottage Restaurant in County Cork. The purée is based on a thick béchamel sauce, which tempers the force of the fennel. She serves it with lamb and game. It's simple to make and is an idea that can be adapted to fit other vegetables with assertive flavours. If your fennel bulbs are large, then you may need to use all the béchamel sauce. The thing is to taste as you make it, in order to get the balance of flavour just as you like it.

SERVES 6

3 large fennel bulbs
40 g (1½ oz) butter
40 g (1½ oz) plain flour

150 ml (5 fl oz) milk
150 ml (5 fl oz) single cream
Salt and freshly ground black pepper

Trim off the stalks and base of each fennel bulb, then slice thinly. Cook in just enough lightly salted water to cover, until tender. Drain, reserving the water.

Melt the butter in a saucepan and stir in the flour. Cook, stirring, for 1 minute. Gradually mix in the milk and then the cream. Bring up to the boil, stirring, and simmer gently for 5–10 minutes, until the béchamel is very thick. Stir occasionally to prevent catching.

Liquidize the cooked fennel in a mixer with 2–3 tablespoons of its cooking water. Add about two-thirds of the béchamel sauce and whizz until smooth. Taste and, if the fennel flavour is too strong, add a little more of the béchamel. Season with salt and pepper. Re-heat before serving.

Baked Fennel with Parmesan

This is my all-time favourite way to cook fennel. It is about as straightforward as a gratin can be – cooked fennel, dredged with Parmesan and baked until brown and bubbling. A heavenly pairing of flavours. Serve it with good bread as a first course, or as a side dish.

SERVES 4–6
3 large *or* 4 medium-sized fennel bulbs
40 g (1½ oz) butter
Freshly ground black pepper
50 g (2 oz) freshly grated Parmesan
 cheese

Trim the tough stalks off each fennel bulb, slice off the base and discard the outer layer if it is damaged. Quarter the bulbs from top to base. Steam or simmer the fennel in salted water until *al dente*. Drain well.

Pre-heat the oven to gas mark 6, 400°F (200°C). Butter a shallow ovenproof dish large enough to take the fennel in a closely packed single layer. Arrange the fennel in the dish, season with pepper. Dot with butter and sprinkle evenly with Parmesan. Bake, uncovered, in the oven for 20 minutes or so until the cheese is browned. Serve immediately.

Roast Poussins with Fennel

Fennel provides the essential boost that mild-flavoured poussins need if they are to be at all interesting. The fennel is used to flavour not only the birds as they roast but also the sauce that will be served with them.

SERVES 2 generously
1 large fennel bulb
2 poussins
40 g (1½ oz) butter
Salt and freshly ground black pepper

1 tablespoon plain flour
250 ml (8 fl oz) milk
85 ml (3 fl oz) single cream
Freshly grated nutmeg

Pre-heat the oven to gas mark 6, 400°F (200°C).

Trim the fennel, reserving the green leaves, and quarter. Place one quarter inside each poussin, and dice the remaining two quarters finely. Smear the breasts of the poussins with half the butter, and season with salt and pepper. Sit in a roasting tin and roast for 30–40 minutes until cooked through.

While they cook, melt the remaining butter and add the diced fennel (but not the fronds). Stir, then cover and sweat over a low heat for 15 minutes. Remove lid and sprinkle in the flour. Cook for 1 minute, stirring. Gradually add the milk a little at a time, stirring well, to make a smooth sauce. Add the cream. Bring to the boil and simmer gently for 5–8 minutes, stirring occasionally. Season with salt, pepper and nutmeg to taste.

If not serving immediately spear a small knob of cold butter on a fork and rub over the surface of the sauce to prevent a skin forming. Just before serving, re-heat the sauce adding a little extra milk if it seems over-thick when warmed through. Stir in the fennel fronds. Serve with the poussins.

Fennel Salad

This salad is so simple that I'm not giving quantities. As a rough guide, one fennel bulb should be enough to feed three to four people depending on its size. It may not look like a huge amount, but raw fennel has a strong taste. As a first course this salad goes very well with thinly sliced bresaola or air-dried ham – such as Parma ham or jamon serrano – and good bread.

> Fennel bulb(s)
> Lemon juice
> Olive oil
> Salt and freshly ground black pepper
> Chopped fresh parsley to garnish

Trim the fennel, removing tough stalks and base, but reserving the green feathery fronds. Quarter, then slice each quarter very, very thinly. Arrange slices in a serving dish, squeeze over lemon juice, then a generous drizzle of olive oil. Season with salt and pepper. Chop the reserved fronds roughly and scatter over the top, along with a little chopped parsley.

ROOTS

Potatoes • Carrots
Beetroot • Turnips • Parsnips
Jerusalem Artichokes

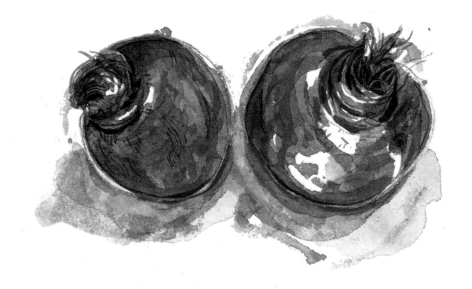

Potatoes

Youghal is a pleasant seaside town in County Cork with no obvious signs of its special place in the history of Ireland and the British Isles. It was here that the potato got its first proper foothold in our islands, when Sir Walter Raleigh planted them on his estate towards the end of the sixteenth century. A few years earlier, Sir John Hawkins had tried growing potatoes in Britain, but they were not a success – they may possibly have been sweet potatoes which need a hot climate. After Sir Walter Raleigh's experiments, potatoes gradually caught on in Ireland. By the middle of the next century they were already a staple crop there, though it took much longer for them to become universally popular in England, Wales and Scotland.

Four hundred years later, it is hard to believe that potatoes were ever considered a dangerous and unhealthy crop (they were even suspected of causing leprosy). They are now the world's most widely grown vegetable and we take it for granted that there will always be plentiful supplies of cheap potatoes.

In recent years, the potato has taken on high fashion status in the food world. At last, the shopper and the gardener are being offered a wide range of potato varieties, from main-crops to new, waxy to floury. New varieties are being developed all the time and, thanks to the current culinary interest, there's an increased emphasis on flavour as well as disease resistance and yield. UK Champion Potato Grower Charles Maisey introduced me to half a dozen or so potatoes that he is trialling for major seed merchants. His favourite is the Kestrel with a delicious buttery taste and slightly waxy texture. With luck it will soon be hitting the markets, having made it through the trials with flying colours.

Stoved Potatoes with Garlic and Coriander

Slowly cooked in olive oil, stoved potatoes are meltingly tender. The whole cloves of garlic not only give flavour, but soften and mellow to a mild sweetness. This is a lovely way to cook both new and old potatoes.

SERVES 3–4

450 g (1 lb) new potatoes or waxier
   main-crop potatoes (e.g. Cara)
1 head of garlic

Salt and freshly ground black pepper
3 tablespoons olive oil
2 tablespoons chopped fresh coriander

Preparing Potatoes

Each year I look forward to the first appearance of Jersey Royals, the unassailable kings of new potatoes, so good that I would never dream of doing anything but steam or boil them with sprigs of mint. Like all new potatoes, they should be bought in small quantities. New potatoes kept hanging around may look fine, but they will have an unpleasant mouldy taste that makes them quite inedible.

Main-crop potatoes are the ones that keep well, as long as they are in good condition to start with. That means no holes or cuts or rotting patches. They should be stored in a cool, mildly humid dark place with a maximum temperature of 50°F/10°C but no colder than 45°F/7°C. Don't keep potatoes in the fridge. The starches will convert to sugar which spoils the flavour – though if they are then left in a warm room for 4 or 5 days the process is usually reversed. Green patches indicate a build up of toxic alkaloids called solanines which congregate when the tubers are exposed to too much light. You can still use the potatoes, but remove all green patches assiduously.

To peel or not to peel? Purely on a time-and-motion basis, I never bother unless there is a particularly good reason for spending time on peeling, eg, for chips. Potatoes cooked in their skins have a better flavour anyway, and they absorb a little less water. Once cooked, the skins come off easily with much less wastage. For the best mash, by the way, you should always leave potatoes unpeeled if you are boiling them, so that they are less watery. Better still bake or microwave them.

Once peeled and cut, potatoes will turn brown if left lying around. Submerging them in water prevents this, but much of their starch will leech out into the water. This is a good thing in some cases – matchstick chips or crisps, for example – where the last thing you want is for them to glue together in clumps in the hot oil. In other recipes, where the starch plays an important role (as a thickener in soups perhaps, or in a gratin), it is not such a good idea. You'll either have to leave preparation until the last minute or put up with slightly discoloured potatoes.

If the new potatoes are very small, leave them as they are. With medium-sized ones, cut in half or quarters. The aim is to get all the chunks about the same size so that they cook evenly. If using main-crop potatoes peel and cut into 2.5–4 cm (1–1½ inch) chunks. Separate all the cloves of garlic and peel, but leave whole.

Put the potatoes and garlic into a heavy frying-pan in a single layer. Don't try to force them in too tightly, because you have to be able to turn them. If you've got a few bits too

OVERLEAF *Stoved Potatoes with Garlic and Coriander*

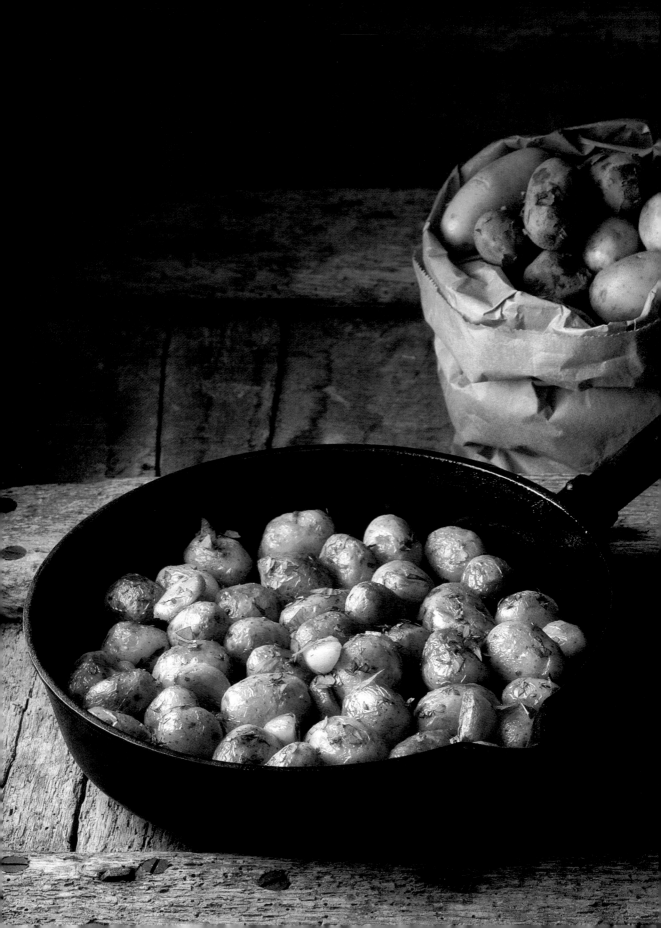

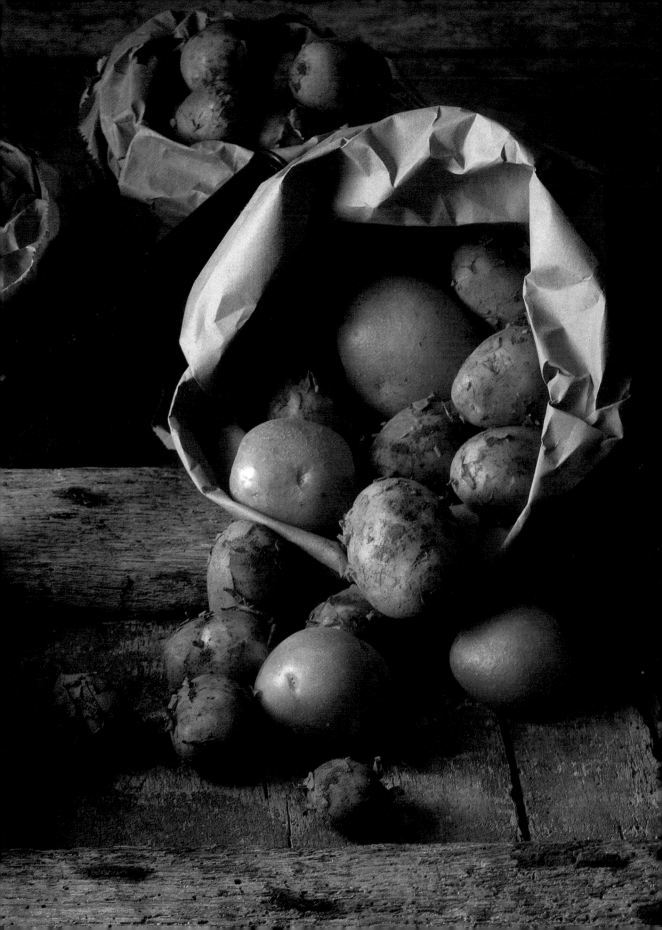

many, then leave them out. Season with salt and pepper, then add 6 tablespoons of water. Drizzle over the olive oil.

Cook, covered, over a low heat for 40 minutes, shaking the pan and stirring occasionally, until potatoes and garlic are very tender and patched with brown. By then the water should have been absorbed. If not, uncover the pan and boil it off. Once they are done, sprinkle over the coriander and serve.

Manuel Socarras' Papas Chorreadas
[Creole Potatoes]

Papas chorreadas is a dish I first tasted in Colombia, but it wasn't until I met Manuel Socarras that I learnt something of its history. Before the Spanish conquest the Colombian Indians used to bury a special kind of potato in bags in the ground, leaving them until they were semi-rotted and imbued with a strange, cheesy flavour. This great delicacy was dished up to the Spaniards who enjoyed the taste but baulked at the theory. Modern-day Papas chorreadas is the conquistadores' version of that ancient dish.

SERVES 6–8

1 generous pinch saffron threads
1 kg (2 lb) red-skinned potatoes
   (e.g. Desirée)

For the sauce
2 tablespoons sunflower oil
1 onion, finely chopped
1 clove garlic, peeled and crushed
1 teaspoon dried thyme
½ teaspoon cumin seeds
225 g (8 oz) tomatoes, skinned,
   de-seeded and chopped

4 spring onions, cut into 5-cm (2-inch)
   pieces and shredded
Salt

1 bay leaf
Salt and freshly ground black pepper
150 g (5 oz) mature Cheddar cheese,
   grated
85 ml (3 fl oz) double cream

Pour a few tablespoons of boiling water over the saffron threads and leave for 10 minutes, stirring occasionally. Place the potatoes in a saucepan with the spring onions, salt and enough water to just cover. Add the saffron and its water to the saucepan together with some salt. Bring to the boil, then cover and simmer until the potatoes are tender. Drain and arrange on a serving dish. Keep warm if necessary.

While the potatoes are cooking make the sauce. Heat the oil in a frying-pan and fry the onion until lightly browned. Add the garlic, thyme and cumin seeds and fry for 1 minute. Then add the chopped tomatoes, bay leaf, salt and pepper. Cook over a vigorous heat until the tomatoes have broken down to form a thick sauce. Add the cheese and cream and stir until the cheese has melted smoothly into the sauce. Pour over the potatoes and serve immediately.

Manuel Socarras' Ajiaco Bogotano
[Colombian Potato and Chicken Soup]

Ajiaco is a speciality of Bogotá, although variations can be found throughout Colombia and other Latin American countries. It's a delicious, comforting, main course soup, designed for cold nights in the Andes but, with its five relishes and garnishes, just as good for a supper party on a cold British night. It was made for me by Manuel Socarras who, like all Colombians, is a fervent devotee of the potato. Ajiaco must be made with a minimum of three types of potato to provide taste, texture and colour. Back home in Colombia Manuel would always use the tiny, yellow-fleshed Criollo potato which is the national pride and joy, but here he has to make do with waxy salad or new potatoes. He's also short of another essential ingredient, the Colombian herb 'guasca', which is rather like a mentholated oregano. Manuel suggests using a combination of fresh parsley and coriander instead.

SERVES 6–8

1 onion, finely chopped
2 tablespoons sunflower oil
1 clove garlic, peeled and crushed
½ tablespoon dried thyme
4 chicken breasts *or* 8 boned chicken thighs
1 litre (1¾ pints) milk
1 litre (1¾ pints) water
450 g (1 lb) red-skinned potatoes (e.g. Desirée), peeled and diced

450 g (1 lb) white potatoes (e.g. King Edwards), peeled and diced
500 g (1 lb 2 oz) small salad *or* new potatoes, scrubbed and thickly sliced
Salt and freshly ground black pepper
4 heads of corn-on-the-cob, husks and silky threads removed, cut into 5-cm (2-inch) lengths
2 tablespoons fresh coriander, chopped
2 tablespoons fresh parsley, chopped

For the egg salad

1 egg, hard-boiled and finely chopped
1 tablespoon chopped fresh parsley
1 tablespoon chopped fresh coriander

2 tablespoons double *or* soured cream
Salt and freshly ground black pepper

For the hot pepper sauce

1 tablespoon chopped fresh coriander
1 tablespoon chopped fresh parsley
1 spring onion, chopped
1 fresh red *or* green chilli, de-seeded and finely chopped

2 tablespoons white wine vinegar
1 tablespoon olive oil
Salt to taste
Sugar to taste

To serve

5 tablespoons capers
250 ml (8 fl oz) double *or* soured cream
2 ripe avocados

Fry the onion gently in the oil in a large saucepan until tender, without browning. Add the garlic and thyme and fry gently for 1 minute more. Raise the heat and add the chicken pieces. Fry until lightly browned. Add the milk, water, all three types of potato and salt and pepper. Bring to the boil, then reduce heat and simmer, covered, for about 40 minutes. Lift out the chicken pieces and as soon as they are cool enough to handle, shred into small pieces.

Stir the soup with a wooden spoon to help the potatoes break down and thicken the soup. Add the corn-on-the-cob pieces and continue cooking over a medium heat for another 10 minutes or so, stirring from time to time, until the corn is tender. Add the coriander, parsley and shredded chicken, and cook for a further 5 minutes or so. Taste and adjust seasoning.

While the soup is cooking, start preparing the 5 garnishes (egg salad, hot pepper sauce, capers, cream, and avocado). To make the egg salad, mix the chopped egg with the parsley and coriander, cream, and salt and pepper. Spoon into a small bowl.

To make the hot pepper sauce, mix the coriander and parsley with the spring onion and chilli, vinegar, oil, salt and a little sugar. Place in a small bowl.

Put the capers and cream into separate bowls. Just before serving, peel and slice the avocado and arrange on a plate. To serve, place the garnishes in the centre of the table, ladle the soup into deep bowls, and let everyone help themselves to the garnishes.

Baked New Potatoes with Anchovy and Parsley

There's no law to say that new potatoes should only be boiled or steamed. Baking them slowly in the oven gives them a luxurious buttery texture. The anchovy fillets dissolve into the pan juices, without giving an overtly fishy flavour, so the potatoes are good with any main course, fish, meat or vegetable.

SERVES 4–6

1 kg (2 lb) new potatoes	2 cloves garlic, peeled and crushed with
40 g (1½ oz) butter	a little salt
3 tablespoons olive oil	2 tablespoons chopped fresh parsley
3 anchovy fillets, chopped	2 tablespoons lemon juice
	Salt and freshly ground black pepper

Pre-heat the oven to gas mark 6, 400°F (200°C).

Scrub the potatoes, removing as much skin as you can. Halve or quarter larger ones. Pat dry on kitchen paper. In a flameproof roasting tin, heat the butter with the oil. Add the anchovy fillets and cook for a minute or so, mashing the fillets into the oil with a fork. Add the potatoes and fry for 4 minutes until they are beginning to colour. Stir in the garlic and parsley, and pour in 150 ml (5 fl oz) water at arm's length (it's bound to spit back at you). Add the lemon juice, a little salt and plenty of pepper.

Move the tin to the oven and bake the potatoes for 25–30 minutes, stirring and basting every 10 minutes or so, until browned and meltingly tender. Spoon the potatoes into a warm dish and pour the richly flavoured juices in the pan over them. Serve.

Himmel und Erde

Himmel und Erde *means heaven and earth, though the connotations here are not particularly spiritual. It refers to the two main ingredients: apples from up above (i.e. trees) and potatoes from the earth. The Germans are particularly strong on combinations of fruit with savoury ingredients, and this is a favourite of mine.*

SERVES 4 generously

1 kg (2 lb) floury potatoes
450 g (1 lb) cooking apples
Sugar to season

Generous knob of butter
Salt and freshly ground black pepper

Peel the potatoes and cut into chunks. Put in a pan with just enough lightly salted water to cover them. Bring to the boil and simmer until almost cooked. Meanwhile, peel, core and chop the apples roughly.

Pour off about two thirds of the water the potatoes are cooking in, then add the apples and simmer gently until they have collapsed and potatoes are melting. Mash together, and season with salt, pepper and a little sugar. Stir in the butter, then tip into a serving dish and serve.

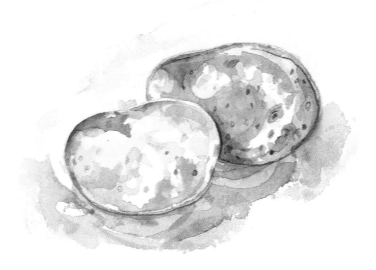

Pommes de Terres Girondines

The Gironde is the wide stretch of water that runs from the Atlantic ocean down almost as far as Bordeaux, fed by two rivers, the Dordogne and the Garonne. It gives its name to the area of land bordering on it. Here you will find the vineyards of many of the great wine-growing châteaux of Bordeaux, but the fertile soil is perfect for growing other produce apart from grapes. The potatoes of Eysines, for instance, a few miles from Bordeaux, are highly rated by the locals.

The curious thing about this method of cooking potatoes, is that they end up with a distinct taste of artichokes. Be that as it may, it is a very easy way to cook the most delicious dish of potatoes, with its hint of garlic, and the mild sharpness of vinegar sizzled in at the end.

SERVES 4

750 g (1¾ lb) potatoes
Salt and freshly ground black pepper
100 g (4 oz) smoked streaky bacon, diced

2 cloves garlic, peeled and halved
2 tablespoons chopped fresh parsley
2 tablespoons white wine vinegar

Peel the potatoes and rinse in cold water. Slice thinly. Find a heavy frying-pan or wide pan, into which the potatoes will just fit neatly. Press the potatoes into the pan, add enough water to half cover, and season lightly with salt. Cover and cook over a fairly high heat, for 12 minutes or so, until the potatoes are just cooked.

Meanwhile, fry the bacon slowly so that it begins to release its own fat. Once there's a thin layer of fat on the base of the pan, add the cloves of garlic. Continue to cook over a gentle heat, until the bacon has given up all its fat and is beginning to brown. Draw off the heat and wait until the potatoes are done.

Once the potatoes are cooked drain off any excess water, and return to the heat. Re-heat the bacon in its fat, until it begins to smoke. Fish out the garlic and discard. Pour bacon and fat evenly over the cooked potatoes, still in their pan and add the parsley, pepper and vinegar. Stir gently to mix, and serve.

Carrots

Carrots aren't always orange. There are white-rooted carrots and yellow-rooted carrots, but the biggest shock of all is coming face-to-face with a purple carrot! Purple carrots have a much longer history than orange ones which were only developed in the Middle Ages. Now they survive only in isolated pockets, one of which is the island of Mallorca. However, you won't find them on restaurant menus – they're strictly for the locals. I brought some home with me, curious to find out what these almost black roots tasted like. Microwaved or steamed, they retain enough of the colour (the purple is only in the outer layers, paling to white in the centre) to cause some bemusement and even consternation at the dining-table. The taste is good, more earthily carroty than orange ones, but much less sweet.

Carrots and islands seem to make interesting bedfellows, in my experience. I flew by helicopter to the Hyskeir lighthouse, standing proud on a tiny island, way out beyond the Isle of Skye. It's one of the last handful of manned lighthouses around Scotland. The three lighthouse keepers work four weeks on and four weeks off and there are few amusements to while away the hours. The truncated golf-course is now overgrown, but the vegetable plot at the base of the lighthouse is still going strong. The main communal plot supplies the lighthouse kitchen, whilst the keepers each have their own personal plot where they grow vegetables to take with them when they return home.

Every single one of the keepers seems to have a passion for carrots. Throughout the year they enjoy their carrots to the full: using the spindly thinnings raw in salads or for dips; savouring them plainly cooked at their optimum middling size; and working their way through the mature fuller-flavoured carrots stored for winter.

Carrot and Mint Salad

If you grow your own carrots, use the slender thinnings to make this salad of fried carrots with mint. If you are not so lucky, then look out for tiny baby carrots, an inch and a half or so long. Failing that, get the smallest carrots you can and cut them into suitably sized pieces.

As the carrots fry slowly in the olive oil, they caramelize on the outside to an intense earthy sweetness. Dressed with lemon juice and plenty of mint, they make an excellent hors d'œuvre.

OVERLEAF *Carrot and Mint Salad*

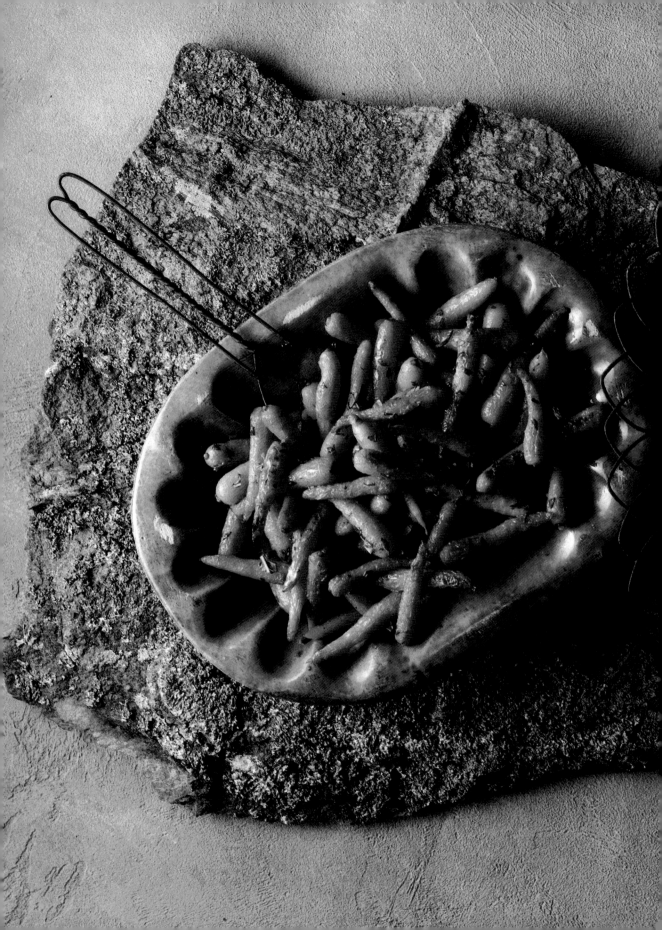

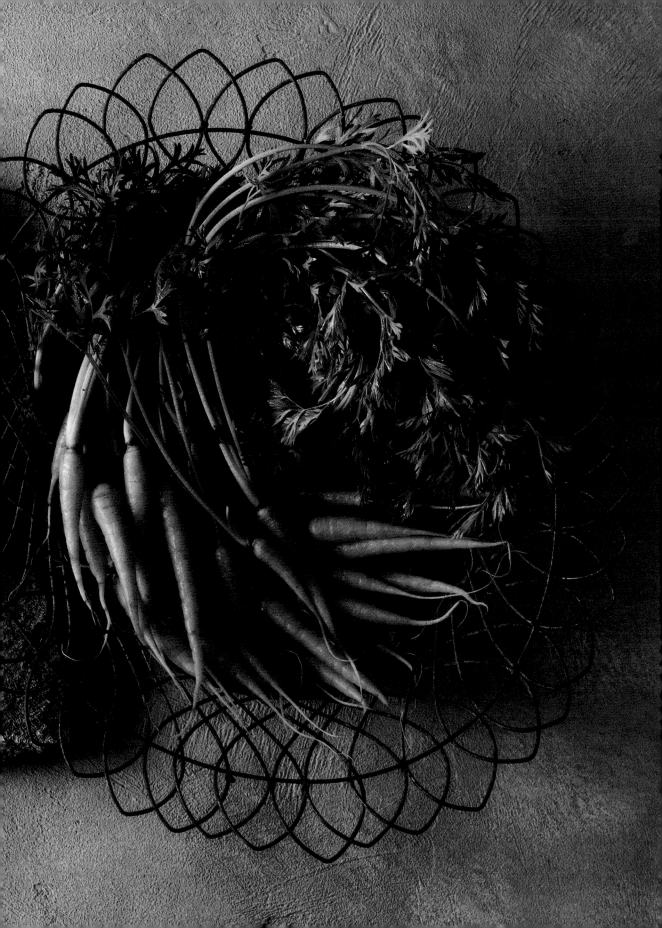

Preparing Carrots

Very young carrots need little preparation other than a good wash to rinse off the dirt. Cook them with a minimum of water, a generous pinch of sugar, a little butter and a dash of lemon juice to enhance their immature flavour. As carrots get older and bigger, they may need to be scraped and, eventually at full size, peeled. I usually nibble a small piece raw to see how large their sugar ration is. If they are sweet and juicy, I will cook them *au nature*, either boiled, again in as little water as I can get away with, or better, steamed. When they are on the dull side, sugar and lemon juice go into the water along with the salt to give them a boost.

Carrots are essential in mixed vegetable soups, adding colour, texture and their much needed sweet flavour. I like grated carrot, too – raw in salads in small quantities (too much makes me feel like a rabbit) with a good mustardy vinaigrette, or cooked with no added water to retain their true full flavour (see opposite). But it is roast carrots, parboiled then browned around a joint of meat, that I like best of all. Seriously big carrots are good for grating and roasting, but really come into their own in stews, where they hold their shape admirably through hours of simmering.

Look out in shops for 'baby' carrots (actually fully mature carrots of a special miniature variety) and the little round extra sweet Paris carrots, more highly priced than the usuals, but worth splashing out on from time to time.

SERVES 4

450 g (1 lb) baby carrots or small carrots
3 tablespoons olive oil
Juice of ½ lemon
2 tablespoons chopped fresh mint
Salt and freshly ground black pepper

If you are using baby carrots, just trim off the tops and any tails. If using small carrots, top and tail, then quarter lengthwise, and cut each piece in half.

Heat the oil in a wide, heavy frying-pan and add the carrots. Fry slowly, shaking and turning every now and then, until the carrots are patched with brown and tender. This should take about 20 minutes. Tip into a bowl and mix with the lemon juice, mint, salt and pepper. Leave to cool and serve at room temperature.

Oded Schwartz's Carrot and Almond Chutney

When master-pickler Oded Schwartz sent a jar of this irresistible chutney into the production office we simply couldn't stop eating it. The jar was passed around and around, with everyone dipping in, until it was all gone. Chutney or chatni, *as it is known in Hindi, originated in India but Oded's chutney is derived from various recipes, including Carrot Halwa, an Indian sweet, and a similar Jewish confection served at Passover. Oded recommends serving it with lamb, or hard, mature cheese. I like it so much I'm perfectly happy to eat it neat.*

MAKES about 2.25 kg (5 lb)

1 kg (2 lb) carrots, peeled
150 g (5 oz) peeled fresh ginger
Finely grated zest and juice of
    2 lemons
5 g (⅛ oz) ground chilli *or* to taste
25 g (1 oz) salt

25 g (1 oz) ground coriander
500 ml (17 fl oz) cider vinegar
300 ml (10 fl oz) water
120 ml (4 fl oz) clear honey
750 g (1½ lb) sugar
60 g (2¼ oz) flaked almonds

Grate the carrots coarsely lengthwise to achieve the longest strands possible. Cut half the ginger into matchsticks and grate the remainder finely. Mix the carrots and all the ginger with the lemon zest and juice, chilli, salt and coriander. Cover with the vinegar and leave overnight.

Transfer the marinated carrots and their juices to a preserving pan and add the water. Bring to the boil and simmer for 20 minutes. Add the honey and sugar and stir to dissolve. Bring back to the boil and boil for 25 minutes or until the mixture is thick. Stir in the almonds and boil for a further 4–5 minutes. Spoon into hot, sterilized jars and seal immediately. The chutney can be eaten straightaway, although it will improve after storing for a few months.

To sterilize jars

Wash in warm soapy water then rinse in hot water. Without touching the insides, set on a wire rack in the oven, set to gas mark ½, 225°F (110°C). Leave for at least half an hour, until the chutney is ready to be potted.

Hot Carrot Shreds

With a food processor to take the knuckle-scraping out of grating, this is one of the quickest ways to cook carrot. With nothing more than a knob of butter and their own juices to sweat in, the flavour is intense and rich. Vary by adding herbs or peeled and grated fresh ginger if you wish, but it isn't really necessary.

SERVES 2

25 g (1 oz) butter
350 g (12 oz) carrots, peeled and
    coarsely grated

Salt and freshly ground black pepper
Squeeze of lemon juice

Melt the butter in a saucepan and add the carrots and a little salt and pepper. Stir to coat evenly, then cook gently for about 5 minutes half-covered, stirring occasionally, until the carrots are tender. Add a squeeze of lemon juice and serve.

Carrot and Tarragon Purée

Puréed carrots take on the most remarkable, almost fluorescent, orange colour. The taste isn't at all bad either and a hint of tarragon points up the flavour neatly. Serve the purée as a side dish with roast chicken or feathered game, or with plainly cooked fish.

SERVES 4

450 g (1 lb) carrots, peeled and sliced
100 g (4 oz) floury potatoes, peeled and
    cut into chunks
½ teaspoon sugar
½ tablespoon lemon juice

1 teaspoon chopped fresh tarragon
    or ½ teaspoon dried
Salt and freshly ground black pepper
25 g (1 oz) butter
Chopped fresh parsley

Put the carrots, potatoes, sugar, lemon juice, tarragon and salt in a pan. Add enough water to cover, bring up to the boil and simmer until vegetables are very tender. Drain, reserving the cooking liquid. Place the vegetables in a food processor with 2 tablespoons of the cooking water. Whizz to a smooth purée, adding more cooking water if necessary. Taste and adjust seasonings. Cool if not serving straight away.

To re-heat the purée, place in a pan with the butter and stir over a moderate heat until piping hot. Pile into a serving bowl and scatter with parsley.

Bœuf à la Mode en Gelée

Bœuf à la mode is the French equivalent of our own boiled beef and carrots. The carrots and beef are cooked separately but they come together, sweet and savoury, in the final dish. Bœuf à la mode is usually served cold, set in its own richly flavoured jelly, but it can be re-heated to serve as a stew. In fact, it's an ideal dinner party or Sunday lunch dish for this country – if the weather turns out warm, eat it cold, but if there's an unexpected nip in the air, eat it hot and steaming.

SERVES 6–8

1.5–1.75 kg (3–4 lb) piece of topside
75 g (3 oz) streaky bacon, cut into strips
3 tablespoons oil
3 tablespoons brandy
1 large onion, chopped
2 stalks celery, sliced
2 cloves garlic, peeled and halved
750 g (1½ lb) carrots, peeled and
    thinly sliced

2 pigs trotters
4 allspice berries
2 bay leaves
2 large sprigs of fresh thyme
1 sprig of fresh rosemary
3 sprigs of fresh parsley
600 ml (1 pint) red wine
900 ml–1.2 litres (1½–2 pints) beef stock
Salt and freshly ground black pepper

Bard the beef with the bacon (i.e. make holes in the beef and push the strips deep down into it). Pat dry, and then brown in the oil. Move to a deep, snug casserole dish. Warm the brandy, set alight and pour over the beef. Once the flames have gone out, add the onion, celery, garlic, 100 g (4 oz) of the carrots, the trotters, spices and herbs. Pour over the wine and enough beef stock to come three-quarters of the way up the beef. Bring gently to the boil, cover and simmer very gently for about 4 hours, turning the beef occasionally. Once it is done, scoop out enough of the stock to cook the remaining carrots in, then leave the beef to cool for 2–3 hours in the remaining stock.

Cook the carrots in the reserved stock, seasoning lightly with salt and pepper, then cool in the stock. Strain, reserving stock and carrots separately. Tear the beef into shreds. Strain its stock and mix with the carrot stock, then boil until reduced to 600 ml (1 pint). Taste and adjust seasoning. Line a bowl with about half of the carrots. Pack in the meat and remaining carrots. Pour over the stock. Leave overnight in the fridge to set. Just before serving, dip the bowl in hot water for a few seconds to loosen, then turn out onto a serving plate. Slice with a sharp knife.

Chicken (or Lamb) and Carrot Tagine

This is a Moroccan dish of aromatically spiced chicken and carrots. A tagine is a special cooking dish, wide and shallow with a conical lid. The exotic stews that are cooked in it have taken on the name of the dish itself. Unless you own a proper tagine, use the widest pan you have.

SERVES 4–6

1 large chicken *or* 1 kg (2 lb) stewing lamb
2 onions, chopped
1½ teaspoons ground ginger
¼ teaspoon saffron threads
5-cm (2-inch) stick of cinnamon
1 clove garlic, peeled and chopped
Freshly ground black pepper

1 teaspoon salt
3 tablespoons olive oil
1 kg (2 lb) carrots, peeled and thickly sliced
3 tablespoons chopped fresh parsley
3 tablespoons chopped fresh coriander
1 tablespoon runny honey
Squeeze of lemon juice

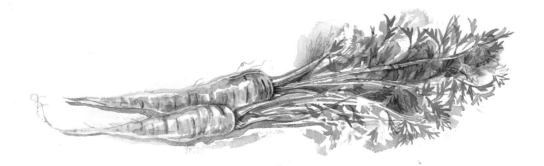

Cut the chicken into 8 pieces. If using lamb, cut into 4-cm (1½-inch) cubes. Place meat, 1 chopped onion, spices, garlic, pepper, salt and oil in a wide flameproof casserole or heavy saucepan. Add enough water to just cover. Cover, bring to the boil and simmer gently.

After 50 minutes, or when the meat is almost cooked, add the remaining onion, carrots and 2 tablespoons each of parsley and coriander, and the honey. Stir and continue simmering, uncovered, for a further 30–40 minutes until the liquid is reduced to a thick, syrupy sauce. Stir in a generous squeeze of lemon juice.

Adjust seasonings and serve, sprinkled with the remaining parsley and coriander.

Boulestin's Ragout of Carrots

Many, many years ago, back in the 1930s X. Marcel Boulestin wrote the Evening Standard *cookery column. Not long after I began to write the same column in the 1980s a bookseller sent me a copy of Boulestin's* The Evening Standard Book of Menus. *The recipes are delightful, showing no signs of over fifty years' wear and tear. This ragout of carrots has certainly withstood the test of time, a good accompaniment to any meal.*

SERVES 4

450 g (1 lb) carrots	Salt and freshly ground black pepper
1 tablespoon lemon juice	1½ tablespoons butter
Bouquet garni (see p. 36)	1 tablespoon plain flour
Pinch of nutmeg	

Scrape the carrots and cut them diagonally into thin slices. Bring 600 ml (1 pint) of water to the boil and add the lemon juice, bouquet garni, nutmeg, salt and pepper. Add the carrots and simmer until they are just tender. Remove the carrots with a slotted spoon, and boil the liquid hard until it is reduced by half.

Melt 1 tablespoon of the butter in a saucepan and mix in the flour. Cook for 1 minute without browning. Remove from the heat and add the reduced cooking water from the carrots little by little to make a white sauce. Bring to the boil and simmer for a further 5 minutes. Taste, adjust seasonings, and stir in the carrots. Heat through thoroughly then, off the heat, stir in the remaining butter. Serve immediately.

Beetroot

A lot of people hate beetroot. Or at least, they think they do, but they've probably never tasted it as it should be. Beetroot is actually one of the best of all vegetables, with a sweet, earthy unique flavour. I love it, and it infuriates me that it gets such a rotten deal in this country. What contorted reasoning has convinced commerce that swamping beetroot in a lake of malt vinegar is a good thing? No wonder so many people shove it to the side of their plate in disgust.

I won't buy ready-cooked beetroot. It upsets me too much. Besides, fresh beetroot is easy enough to cook. It just takes a bit of time, but the result is ample reward. I've made several beetroot converts in my time, and I'm hoping for more.

Gardeners who grow their own beetroot will need no convincing. One such is fellow beetroot devotee, Matthew Fort, the *Guardian*'s food editor. He started growing beetroot because it was impossible to buy them any smaller than cannonball size. Neat rows of beetroot leaves (which can, incidentally, be eaten like spinach), crowd the raised vegetable plot at the foot of his garden. He pulls the beetroot when they are no more than golf-ball size. Such small, delicately flavoured beetroot needs only to be boiled until just tender and served whole, dressed with butter and herbs, or a light vinaigrette – a true gardener's delight. As well as ordinary purple spherical beetroot, Matthew also grows the pretty yellow-fleshed variety, and when he can get the seeds, white and carrot-rooted beetroot too. It's only when he's making his version of Borshch (p. 67) that he buys in the cannonballs.

Beetroot and Orange Salad

Peel a couple of oranges right down to the flesh. Slice with a sharp knife, and arrange on a plate. Spoon over a little vinaigrette. Dice beetroot, toss in vinaigrette (see p. 177–8) and pile in the centre of the orange slices. Sprinkle with chopped parsley and serve.

Beetroot and Walnut Salad

Toss cubed or sliced beetroot in vinaigrette (see p. 177–8) and place in a dish. Scatter with chopped parsley or chives and toasted walnuts.

Preparing Beetroot

The average-sized, shop-bought beetroot can be cooked in several ways, but is best baked in the oven. Begin by washing it gently. Never scrub a beetroot, or you will break the skin and the purple juices will 'bleed'. Don't break off the root either, for the same reason. Trim the stalks to about 2.5 cm (1 inch) above the beetroot.

Place the prepared beetroot in a close-fitting ovenproof dish and add a couple of tablespoons of water to prevent it drying out. Cover tightly with foil and bake in a low oven (around gas mark 2, 300°F (150°C) for 3–4 hours until the skin wrinkles and is easily scraped away from the root end.

If you haven't got that much time to wait for your beetroot, they can be boiled instead, though the flavour won't be quite so good. Prepare in exactly the same way and boil for 1½–2 hours. When I'm in a real rush, and I only want to cook a couple of beetroot, I turn to the microwave. Set in a bowl, again with a couple of tablespoons of water and tightly covered with clingfilm, a brace of beetroot should take about 8–10 minutes on full power (turn once or twice). Exact cooking time will, of course, vary with the power of the oven and the size of the beetroot.

Once cooked, the field is wide open. There are umpteen salads to be made – beetroot goes particularly well with dill, soured cream, orange, apple and walnuts. One of my favourite French salads mixes beetroot with vinaigrette and toasted walnuts (see p. 65), but as long as you treat the beetroot with due consideration, there's no end to the possibilities. Don't, however, mix the separate components until the last moment, if at all, unless you happen to like the purple juice streaked messily over everything. I prefer to arrange each main ingredient, individually dressed, separately on a serving plate, so that it all looks beautiful when it is served.

Of course, the remarkable staining power of beetroot can be used to good effect. Glowing magenta Borscht is a prime example, and the colour of beetroot purée is one of its great attributes. An Iranian 'burani' (see p. 113–14) made with cooked beetroot rather than spinach turns the most glorious bright pink. No doubt about it, for flavour and colour there's precious little to beat the much under-rated beetroot.

Beetroot Purée

This is so pretty! Beetroot makes the most beautiful deep pink purée that tastes every bit as good as it looks. I first made it to go with roast pheasant, but it would sit happily alongside any main course that can take its rich earthy taste.

SERVES 4

225–275 g (8–10 oz) cooked, peeled
   beetroot
225 g (8 oz) floury potatoes, peeled and
   cooked
85 ml (3 fl oz) soured cream

1 tablespoon chopped fresh dill
   or 1 teaspoon dried
Salt and freshly ground black pepper
25 g (1 oz) butter

Chop the beetroot and potato roughly. Put them in a food processor together with the soured cream, dill, salt and pepper and whizz until smooth. Taste and adjust seasoning. Re-heat gently with the butter when needed.

Matthew Fort's Ukrainian Borshch

Borshch, or borsht, is really a general name for a whole collection of Eastern European beetroot soups that vary enormously. Borshch can be anything from an elegant, clear ruby consommé (some are made with fermented beetroot juice), to a hearty vegetable soup/stew. Matthew Fort's borshch belongs to the latter group and is based on the recipe for Ukrainian borshch given in the Time Life's The Cooking of Russia. *It can be made even more substantial by adding shreds of cooked beef, game, or sliced, grilled sausages.*

SERVES 8–12

1 onion, chopped
2 cloves garlic, peeled and finely
   chopped
50 g (2 oz) butter
½ large celeriac, peeled and coarsely
   grated
1 large parsnip, peeled and coarsely
   grated
450 g (1 lb) raw beetroot, peeled and
   coarsley grated

4 tomatoes, skinned, de-seeded and
   roughly chopped
½–1 teaspoon sugar
3–5 tablespoons red wine vinegar
2 litres (3½ pints) rich beef stock
Salt and freshly ground black pepper
450 g (1 lb) potatoes, peeled and cut
   into chunks
½ large green cabbage, cored and
   shredded

To garnish
Soured cream
Fresh parsley, roughly chopped

OVERLEAF *Matthew Fort's Ukrainian Borshch*

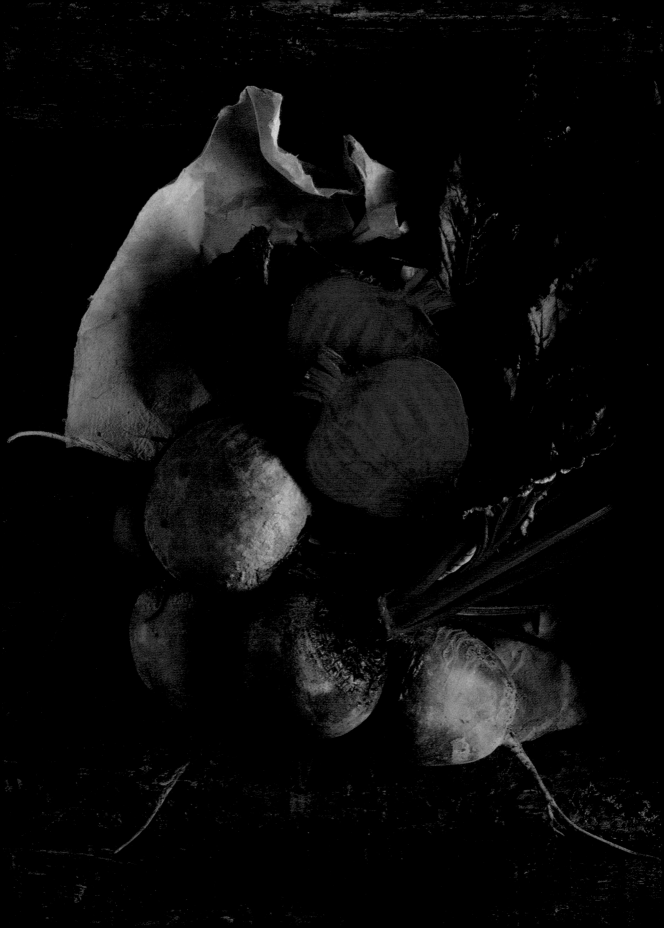

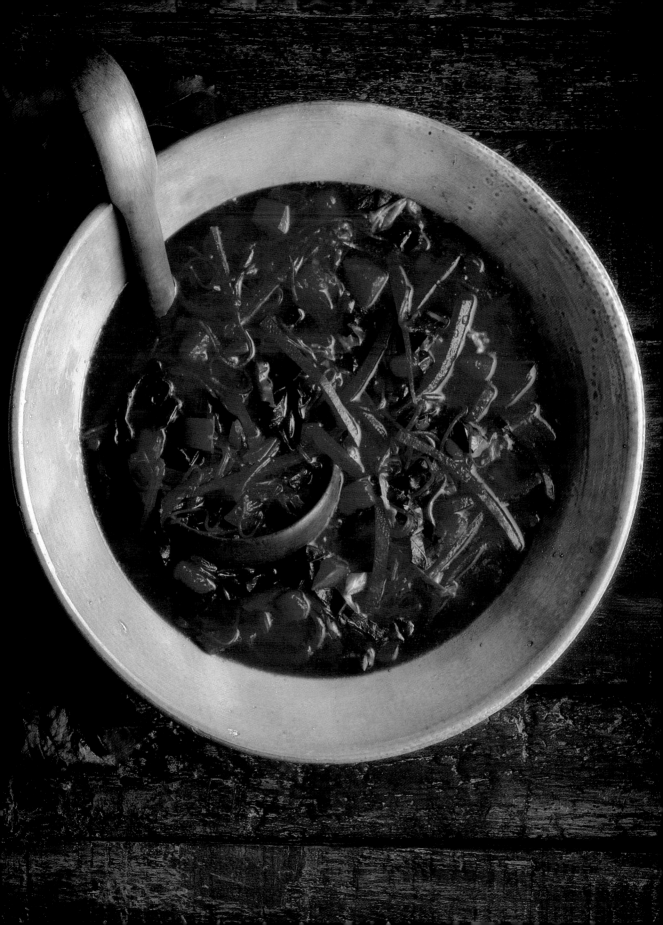

In a large saucepan cook the onion and garlic gently in the butter, without browning, until tender. Add the celeriac, parsnip, beetroot and half the tomatoes. Mix in the sugar, 3 tablespoons of vinegar, a generous 300 ml (10 fl oz) of stock, and salt and pepper. Stir and bring to the boil, then cover and leave to simmer for 40 minutes.

Meanwhile, pour the remaining stock into another large saucepan and bring to the boil. Add the potatoes and cabbage and simmer, half-covered, for 15–20 minutes until the potatoes are tender.

When both pans of vegetables are ready combine them in the largest pan, adding the rest of the tomatoes. Bring back to the boil, simmer for 5–10 minutes, then taste and add a little more seasoning, sugar or vinegar as necessary. Serve in deep soup bowls, topping each bowlful with a dollop of soured cream and a sprinkling of parsley.

Hot Beetroot with Apple

Beetroot and apple go so well together – a starred partnership. The fruity tartness of the fried apple wedges really sets off the earthiness of the beetroot, and the final dressing of horseradish brings the whole lot together neatly.

SERVES 4

2 medium-sized cooked beetroot, peeled	2 tablespoons lemon juice
2 dessert apples	½ teaspoon creamed horseradish
1 tablespoon sunflower oil	Salt and freshly ground black pepper
25 g (1 oz) butter	1½ tablespoons chopped fresh parsley and/or fresh chives

Dice the beetroot into 1-cm (½-inch) cubes. Just before cooking, core and cut the apples into quarters. Cut each quarter in half or thirds, depending on size. Heat the oil and butter in a frying-pan until it foams. Add the apple slices and fry briskly until golden brown. Scoop onto a serving plate, arranging them around the edges. Keep warm.

Add the beetroot cubes to the pan and sauté briefly until hot. Pile them into the centre of the apples and keep warm. Quickly add the lemon juice and horseradish to the pan and stir, scraping in fat and juices. Pour over the beetroot. Season the whole lot with salt and pepper, scatter with herbs, and serve.

Red Flannel Hash

An American classic – corned beef hash with cubes of beetroot. It is not elegant fare, but who cares when it tastes so wonderful. Pile it on to the plate and dig in – you won't be disappointed. If you want to go right over the top, add a fried egg per person, perched on top of the mound of hash.

SERVES 4–6

1 × 350 g (12 oz) tin corned beef, diced
1 onion, finely chopped
450 g (1 lb) cooked potatoes, peeled and
    diced
275 g (10 oz) cooked beetroot, peeled
    and diced

50 g (2 oz) butter
1 tablespoon Worcestershire sauce
Salt and freshly ground black pepper
Freshly chopped fresh parsley

Mix together the corned beef, onion, potatoes, beetroot and a little salt and pepper. If you have the time, leave for a few hours or even overnight, covered, stirring occasionally. This is not essential, but it improves the flavour.

Melt the butter in a wide, heavy frying-pan and heat until it is foaming. Add the corned beef mixture and the Worcestershire sauce. Stir, then press down fairly firmly. Turn the heat down to medium-low and cook gently for about 15 minutes until a brown crust forms on the base. Stir and break up, so that some of the crust gets mixed in with the rest. Add about 4 tablespoons of hot water. Press down again and cook for a further 15 minutes or so, until a second crust has formed. Scoop out on to a dish, scatter with parsley and serve immediately.

Kidneys with Beetroot

I love beetroot and I love kidneys, so when I saw this recipe in Pierre Koffman's autobiographical book La Tante Claire *(Headline Books), I knew it was for me. I've adapted it slightly to fit a domestic kitchen (my local butcher doesn't often have the veal kidneys that Pierre Koffman would use). It is quite superb, a rich and sophisticated way to make use of the humble beetroot.*

SERVES 4

8 lambs kidneys
1 tablespoon sunflower oil
50 g (2 oz) butter
4 shallots, finely chopped
1 medium-cooked beetroot, peeled and
    cut into 5-mm (¼-inch) batons

4 tablespoons dry white wine
120 ml (4 fl oz) chicken *or* veal stock
120 ml (4 fl oz) double cream
2 tablespoons wholegrain mustard
Salt and freshly ground black pepper

Trim the kidneys and cut in half horizontally. Remove core. Heat the oil and half the butter in a wide frying-pan until the butter is foaming. Add the kidneys and sauté until just done. Set them aside and pour any excess fat off from the pan.

Add the remaining butter to the same pan and cook the shallots gently until translucent. Add the beetroot and the white wine and boil until the wine is completely evaporated, leaving just moist beetroot. Quickly add the stock and boil until reduced by half. Then add the cream and boil until the sauce coats the back of a spoon. Whisk in the mustard and return the kidneys to the pan. Warm through gently, seasoning with salt and pepper, and serve immediately.

Turnips

As a child, I found it hard to believe that turnips in France and turnips in England were one and the same vegetable. Everyone assured me that 'navet' meant turnip but, as far as I could see, not only did they look different, but they also tasted very different. I liked 'navets', but I wasn't overly keen on turnips.

I had fair cause for my disbelief. Turnips do come in many shapes and sizes. The ones I'd seen in France were the pretty squashed round type, spattered with a purple blush and small in stature, sometimes very small indeed. English turnips, on the other hand, were big and rather ugly balls, white and green and altogether unprepossessing. Nowadays, my 'French' turnips are much more common in this country, and there are long-rooted turnips around as well.

The difference in taste is easily explained. The French have a serious appreciation for turnips. They cook them lovingly, choosing petite specimens when possible for a more delicate flavour, but they know how to handle their portly and hefty elders to show them at their best. In England we tend to go for the big boys and boil them hard. End of story. Big and overboiled and nothing more is not very fair on poor old turnips. They deserve better, which does not necessarily mean elaborate.

Sautéed Turnips with Cumin and Lemon

A snappy way to give turnips a lift out of the ordinary. Parboiled turnips are quickly fried with cumin and finished with lemon and coriander leaf. Who said turnips were boring?

SERVES 4

450 g (1 lb) turnips
2 tablespoons olive oil
1 teaspoon cumin seeds, crushed
Finely grated zest of ½ lemon
½ tablespoon lemon juice
Salt and freshly ground black pepper
1 tablespoon chopped fresh coriander

Preparing Turnips

In spring, look out for the pretty sight of bunches of glowing quails'-egg-sized turnips with their purply pink cheeks, and long green leaves. These are turnips at their best.

Trim off any leaves (save them), leaving 1 cm (½ inch) or so of greenery sticking up for effect, and steam the turnips which won't need peeling. A knob of butter is enough embellishment, though they can also be glazed (see p. 74) and are perfect for a Navarin printanier (see p. 242–3). Those leaves that you saved can be eaten too, as a spinach-like vegetable boiled until tender, drained and fried for a few minutes over a brisk heat in olive oil or butter.

The next size up, a couple of inches across, will be almost as good, but may need peeling if the skin is already tough. Any bigger and turnips begin to betray their membership of the brassica family, showing signs of one of its least appealing characteristics. There's a definite brassica rankness that creeps into the roots, and it has to be tackled head on.

Peel them, cut them up as appropriate, but before you cook them with any flavourings, blanch them first to draw out the rankness. Four or five minutes in boiling water until they are half-cooked is quite adequate for the job. Drain them, and then they will be fine . . . as long as they are not so very enormous and old and raddled that their flavour defies improvement. As a quick finish, fry them in oil or butter until lightly browned and serve scattered with parsley.

The only time I don't bother with blanching is when they are going, in relatively small quantity, into a stew of some sort. The rank flavour disperses in the cooking liquid and disappears effectively in the mêlée of ingredients, leaving the pieces of turnips with their true, happy character intact.

If the turnips are on the large side, peel and cut into 2-cm (¾-inch) cubes. If they are small spring turnips, just trim and quarter. Drop into a pan of lightly salted boiling water and simmer for 5 minutes until almost, but not quite, cooked. Drain and run under the cold tap. Drain thoroughly and pat dry on kitchen paper.

Heat the oil in a wide frying-pan. Add the cumin seeds and stir for about 30 seconds. Now add the turnips and fry until nicely browned. Stir in the lemon zest and juice, plenty of pepper and a little salt. Turn into a serving dish and scatter with the coriander. Serve.

Ginger-glazed Turnips

I'm not taken with ginger wine as a drink, but it is a great cooking ingredient. In this recipe it gives the turnips a subtle gingery glaze. If you have very small turnips leave them whole. The same method can be used very successfully for carrots.

SERVES 4

450 g (1 lb) medium-sized turnips, peeled and cut into 1-cm (½-inch) cubes	2 tablespoons ginger wine
	Squeeze of lemon juice
	1 tablespoon caster sugar
40 g (1½ oz) butter	Salt and freshly ground black pepper

Cook the turnip cubes in salted boiling water for 2–3 minutes or until almost tender. Drain and run under the cold tap. Drain thoroughly.

Melt the butter in a frying-pan and add the turnips. Fry for a minute or so. Add the remaining ingredients and stir over a medium heat until the turnip cubes are glazed with a rich syrup. Serve immediately.

Spiced Turnips and Chickpeas

This is adapted from a Moroccan recipe for a tagine of lamb, turnips and chickpeas. I've jettisoned the lamb but kept the original blend of aromatic spices and the honey sweetener. It is still substantial enough to work as a main course, served over a bed of couscous or rice.

SERVES 4

175 g (6 oz) dried chickpeas, soaked overnight	1 teaspoon ground cinnamon
1 onion, coarsely grated	1 teaspoon ground ginger
25 g (1 oz) unsalted butter	1 teaspoon ground cumin
1 tablespoon sunflower oil	½ tablespoon ground coriander
750 g (1½ lb) medium-sized turnips, peeled and cut into 1-cm (½-inch) cubes	1 tablespoon honey
	2 tablespoons chopped fresh coriander
	Salt and freshly ground black pepper

Drain the chickpeas and cook in unsalted water until almost but not quite tender. Drain, reserving the cooking water. Blanch the turnips for 2 minutes in boiling water, then drain.

Melt the butter and oil in a wide saucepan and add the chickpeas, onion, turnips, spices and enough of the water from cooking the chickpeas to just cover. Cover and simmer for 15 minutes. Uncover and stir in the honey, half the chopped coriander, salt and plenty of pepper. Simmer, uncovered, for a further 10–15 minutes until the liquid is reduced to a thick sauce. Sprinkle with the remaining coriander and serve.

Root Vegetable Pie

This sturdy root vegetable pie wrapped in puff pastry makes a magnificent main course without breaking the bank. It's one of those recipes that somehow seems to exceed the sum of its parts, tasting ten times better than you might expect. As long as you drain the vegetables thoroughly, the pie can be constructed a couple of hours in advance, and whipped into the oven an hour or so before you plan to eat.

SERVES 4–6

450 g (1 lb) carrots, peeled and sliced
450 g (1 lb) potatoes, peeled and sliced
225 g (8 oz) turnips, peeled and sliced
50 g (2 oz) butter plus extra for greasing tin
450 g (1 lb) puff pastry, thawed if frozen

Flour for rolling out
2 tablespoons finely chopped fresh parsley
2 teaspoons caraway seeds
Salt and freshly ground black pepper
1 egg, beaten

Bring a large pan of lightly salted water to the boil. Cook the carrot slices for about 6 minutes, then scoop out and drain. Repeat with potatoes and turnips, keeping each vegetable separate.

Butter a loose-bottomed cake tin, 5 cm (2 inches) deep by 20 cm (8 inches) in diameter. Roll out two-thirds of the pastry on a lightly floured board to give a rough circle of about 33 cm (13 inches) in diameter. Loosely fold in half and then in quarters, then lift into the tin with the centre tip of the pastry at the centre of the tin. Carefully unfold, then lift the edges and gently push the pastry down to line the sides of the tin using a small knob of pastry rolled into a ball to ease it right into the corner.

Make separate layers of potatoes, carrots, and turnips, sprinkling parsley, caraway seeds, salt and pepper between layers and dotting with butter as you go. Roll out remaining pastry, and lay over the pie. Trim off excess and press the edges of the pastry together firmly. Make a hole in the centre, then let it rest for 30 minutes in the fridge. Pre-heat the oven to gas mark 7, 425°F (220°C).

Brush the top of the pie with beaten egg and bake for 10 minutes until golden brown. Then reduce the heat to gas mark 4, 350°F (180°C) and cook for a further 50–60 minutes. Test with a skewer to check that the vegetables are cooked and tender. Unmould carefully and serve hot or warm.

Parsnips

There's a firmly held belief that parsnips should not be eaten until after the first heavy frosts of late autumn. They always used to be a winter crop, though now we can buy them all the year round, albeit at an inflated price in summer. Small summer parsnips can taste just as good as the massive winter roots, so I'm afraid the frost is no longer an essential element in parsnip cultivation. It is true, however, that cold has a beneficial effect on parsnips, intensifying their sweetness, but you don't need to leave them out on a cold night. A day or two in the fridge will do the trick.

For all that, I do cook and eat far more parsnips in the winter than I ever do in summer. Soft and sweetly flavoured, they are one of those lovely comfort foods that seem so necessary when the weather is chilly and the temperature drops. Unless I intend to stuff them, I usually opt for middling-sized roots harvested before the fibres become tough and stringy and the core too woody to eat. It's always a good idea to inspect parsnips carefully before you buy if you can. Check that they are sound and firm. Once a parsnip begins to show signs of brown rot, it generally means that the whole root is past using and will have to go into the bin.

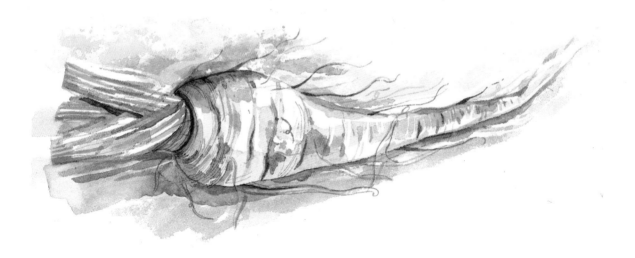

Preparing Parsnips

If parsnips are very small and tender, you may not even need to scrape them before cooking. Once the girth increases they will probably need to be peeled at some stage, before or after cooking. Only with enormous parsnips should you bother to remove the core – more easily done when the parsnip is partially cooked.

For most dishes, the parsnips will need to be par-cooked to some degree first. Be attentive as parsnips soften more quickly than, say, carrots. They should not be done to the extent that they are soft and fuzzy when there's a second stage of cooking to follow, unless you are going to purée them, of course. Cooking them in their skins helps to keep their shape, but remember to peel them afterwards.

Parsnips are low in calories, but they do benefit from some kind of lubrication. Boiled or steamed, they are vastly improved by a generous knob of butter melting over them as they are served. I often boil them until almost done, then finish by frying in a mixture of butter and oil until patched with brown. Toasted chopped hazelnuts or sesame seeds go well with parsnips.

Parsnips make irresistible chips (see p. 78) and are wonderful roast around the joint (in both cases, boiled first until half-cooked). Though they are not an Indian vegetable, I like them a great deal in curries such as the korma on p. 82, where they absorb the flavour of the spices willingly, contributing their own sweet softness in return.

Parsnip Purée

It's not worth giving quantities here. If you can mash potatoes, then you can mash parsnips. The balance of parsnip to potato is very much an individual taste. The potato gives a smoother texture and softens the potentially insistent taste of the parsnip. I usually use roughly half potatoes and half parsnips, but for a stronger sweeter flavour increase the parsnips as you like.

Parsnips	Freshly grated nutmeg *or* ground
Potatoes	cinnamon
Butter	Salt and freshly ground black pepper
Milk *or* single cream	

Peel and chop the potatoes and parsnips roughly. Cook in boiling salted water. Drain thoroughly, and return to the pan. Add a large knob of butter, and start mashing over a low heat. Gradually mash in enough milk or cream to give a creamy purée. Season with nutmeg or cinnamon, and plenty of salt and pepper. Serve.

Fried Parsnips with Walnuts

This is a damn-the-calories way with parsnips. The parsnips are sautéed in butter with walnuts, then finished with sugar and a dash of vinegar to balance. Great with roast game or with hot ham.

SERVES 4

450 (1 lb) small parsnips
15 g (½ oz) light muscovado sugar
¼ teaspoon cinnamon
40 g (1½ oz) butter
25 g (1 oz) walnuts, chopped
1 tablespoon white wine vinegar
Salt and freshly ground black pepper
Chopped fresh parsley to garnish

Peel the parsnips and cook in lightly salted boiling water until almost tender. Drain well, cut each one in half, and then cut the thicker part into quarters lengthwise. Mix the sugar with the cinnamon.

Melt the butter in a wide pan and add the parsnips and walnuts. Fry gently, stirring and turning, until the parsnips are lightly patched with brown. Scatter with sugar and cinnamon, stir to distribute evenly, then drizzle over the vinegar and salt and pepper. Cook for a final minute and serve, scattered with parsley.

Saratoga Chips

Or in other words, parsnip chips. The only difference between making potato chips and parsnip chips, is that the parsnips should be parboiled before they are deep-fried. The real difference lies in the taste.

SERVES 4

1 kg (2 lb) parsnips
Oil for deep-frying
Salt

Cut the parsnips into 5-cm (2-inch) lengths. Quarter the larger ends and remove the woody core. Parboil the parsnip pieces until half-cooked. Drain thoroughly and pat dry on kitchen paper. Deep-fry until golden brown. Drain briefly on kitchen paper and sprinkle with salt. Serve.

Poor Man's Lobster

Or in other words, parsnip salad. Parsnips have always been considered rather lowly vegetables – presumably smart but misleading names, like Poor Man's Lobster, were given to parsnip dishes to disguise their humble nature.

Be that as it may, cooked parsnips are a pleasing addition to winter salads – though they don't bear that much of a relation to pricey lobster. Toss them in vinaigrette (see p. 177–8) while still warm and leave to cool. Serve on a bed of lettuce, with tomato, fresh herbs, quarters of hard-boiled eggs, shrimps, or whatever seems appropriate and is to hand.

Stuffed Parsnips with Sunflower Seeds

Brutally big end-of-season parsnips can seem daunting, but they are just what you need for this recipe. The toughened core goes out, leaving a neat hole to fill up – just begging for a well-flavoured stuffing like the one below. Though the stuffed parsnips could be served as a side dish, I prefer to feature them as a main course, adding a home-made tomato sauce to bolster them up into prominence.

SERVES 4

750 g (1½ lb) large parsnips
1 onion, chopped
1–2 cloves garlic, peeled and chopped
1½ tablespoons finely chopped fresh
    parsley
50 g (2 oz) butter *or* 4 tablespoons
    sunflower oil

100 g (4 oz) breadcrumbs, white
    or brown
15 g (½ oz) sunflower seeds
½ tablespoons fresh thyme leaves
    or chopped fresh rosemary
    or ½ teaspoon dried
Finely grated zest and juice of ½ lemon
Salt and freshly ground black pepper

Peel the parsnips and trim off the tops. Chop the lower thinner parts finely (where the parsnip thins down to less than 4 cm (1½ inches) across). Slice the wider parts into 2.5-cm (1-inch) thick rings. Using an apple corer or a small sharp knife, cut out the woody core. Blanch the rings in boiling salted water for 5 minutes. Drain well and arrange in a single layer in a greased shallow ovenproof dish.

Fry the onion, garlic and chopped parsnips slowly in 40 g (1½ oz) of the butter or 3 tablespoons of the oil until tender. Mix in all of the remaining ingredients. Taste and adjust seasoning.

Pre-heat the oven to gas mark 6, 400°F (200°C). Fill the holes in the parsnip rings with the stuffing, mounding it up over the individual rings. Dot with the remaining butter, or drizzle over the remaining oil. Bake for 25–30 minutes until golden brown. Serve.

OVERLEAF *Stuffed Parsnips with Sunflower Seeds*

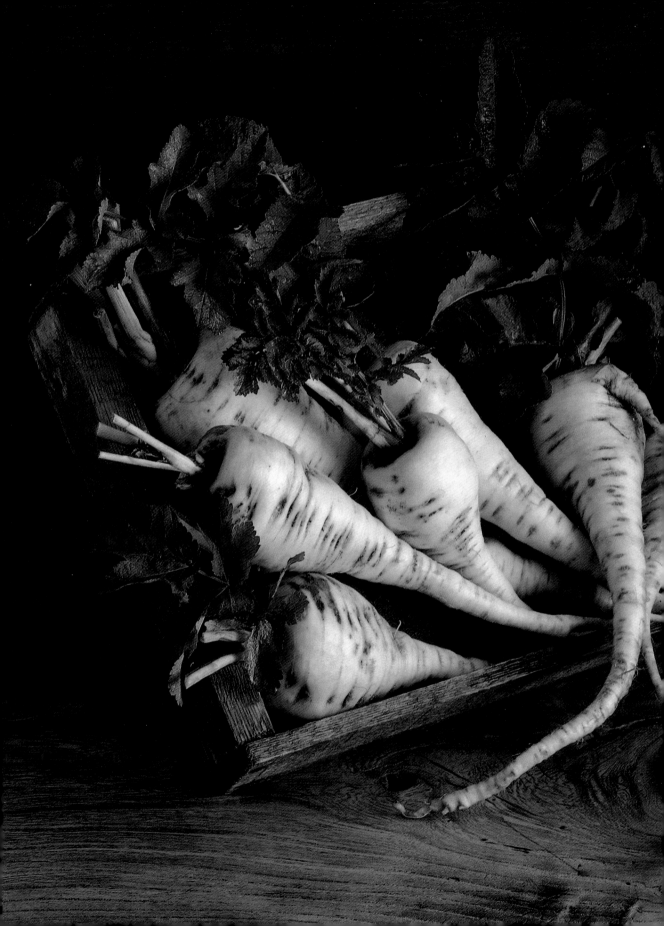

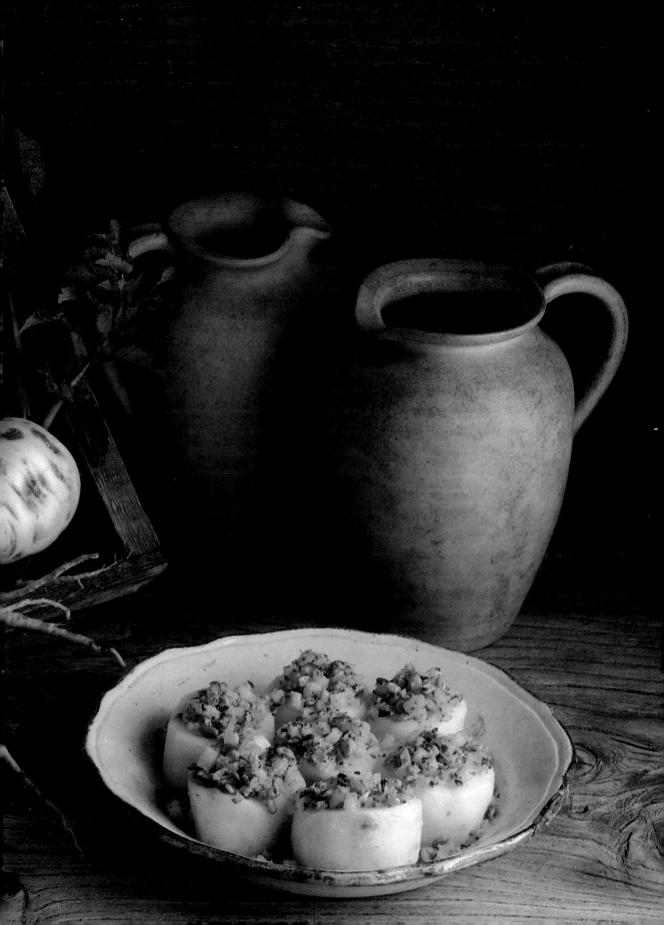

Parsnip, Carrot and Cauliflower Korma

This is a mild but warmly spiced curry, thickened with yoghurt and ground almonds. I usually make it with a mixture of parsnip, carrot and cauliflower, three different flavours and textures. Of course, you can adapt it to practically whatever vegetables you have to hand, as long as you add those that take less time to cook 5 or 10 minutes or so after the slow cooking root vegetables.

Serve with rice, of course, and several relishes: mango chutney, sour lime pickles, and the fresh onion chutney on page 91.

SERVES 4

275 g (10 oz) parsnips
350 g (12 oz) carrots
1 medium onion, finely chopped
4 tablespoons sunflower oil
1 tablespoon ground cumin
2 teaspoons ground coriander
1 teaspoon ground cinnamon
1 teaspoon turmeric
2 cloves garlic, peeled and very finely chopped

2.5-cm (1-inch) piece fresh ginger, peeled and very finely chopped
1 fresh green chilli, de-seeded and very finely chopped
300 ml (10 fl oz) Greek-style yoghurt
40 g (1½ oz) ground almonds
Salt
275 g (10 oz) small cauliflower florets
Finely chopped fresh coriander *or* parsley to garnish

Peel the parsnips and carrots if necessary, and cut in 1-cm (½-inch) slices. If they are large then cube them.

In a saucepan large enough to take all the ingredients fry the onion in the oil until golden brown. Stir in all the dry spices and when well mixed add the garlic, ginger and chilli. Stir gently for 1 minute. Stir in the yoghurt, a tablespoonful at a time and then add the almonds. Cook, stirring, for 2 more minutes.

Stir in 300 ml (10 fl oz) of water and some salt, then add the parsnips, carrots and cauliflower. Cover and simmer gently for 20–25 minutes until the vegetables are almost done, stirring occasionally. Uncover and simmer for a final 5 minutes or so. Taste and adjust seasonings. Sprinkle with coriander or parsley before serving.

Jerusalem Artichokes

One thing is certain about Jerusalem artichokes. They have nothing whatsoever to do with Jerusalem, nor for that matter with artichokes proper. They come, in fact, from North America where they have long been a staple of native Indian tribes. Cherokee Indians call them *gu-ge* and still use them to make relishes, while the traditional way of cooking them was roasted in the embers like baked potatoes.

When the Frenchman, Samuel de Champlain, first came across these Indian tubers at Cape Cod in 1605, he described them as having 'the taste of artichokes' (I think there is a passing resemblance in flavour, but others disagree) and from that likeness they acquired the second part of their name.

The 'Jerusalem' part of this vegetable's name is harder to explain. There are two hypotheses that I've come across and neither can be proved beyond doubt. The one I like best is that botanists realized that the tubers were related to the sunflower, called 'girasole' in Italian. In England, 'girasole' was soon corrupted into 'Jerusalem'. The second possibility is that they were introduced to England from the Netherlands where they had been known as the 'artichoke-apple of Ter Neusen' (a town in the Netherlands) and that it was 'Ter Neusen', not 'girasole' that was corrupted.

Jerusalem Artichokes are, it must be said, notorious for one thing which is not normally discussed in polite society. They make you fart. This doesn't worry me that much, certainly not enough to stop me eating what I think is a most delicious vegetable. For most people there is a delay of at least a couple of hours before wind makes its presence known, quite enough time to finish the meal and withdraw before the onslaught if needs be.

Jerusalem Artichokes with Bacon, Paprika and Breadcrumbs

The salt of the bacon and the crispness of the breadcrumbs set off the tender, sweet Jerusalem artichokes perfectly. I usually keep this as a separate course all on its own. Pancetta is an Italian form of bacon, with a particularly good flavour for cooking. It is available from Italian delicatessens, but if you can't get it use streaky bacon instead. Vegetarians shouldn't ignore this recipe altogether – sliced mushrooms make a good substitute for the bacon.

OVERLEAF *Jerusalem Artichokes with Bacon, Paprika and Breadcrumbs*

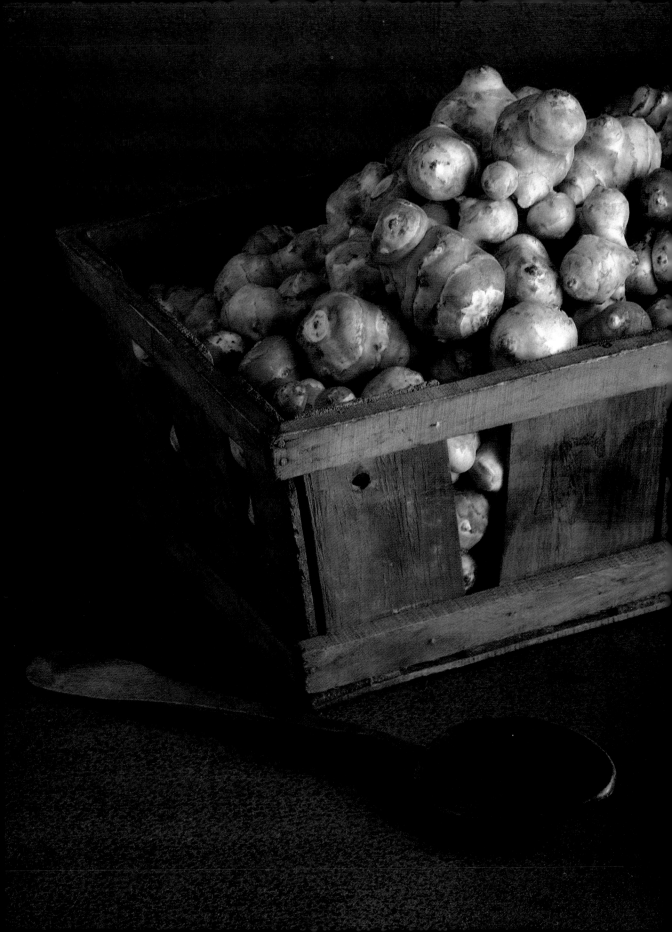

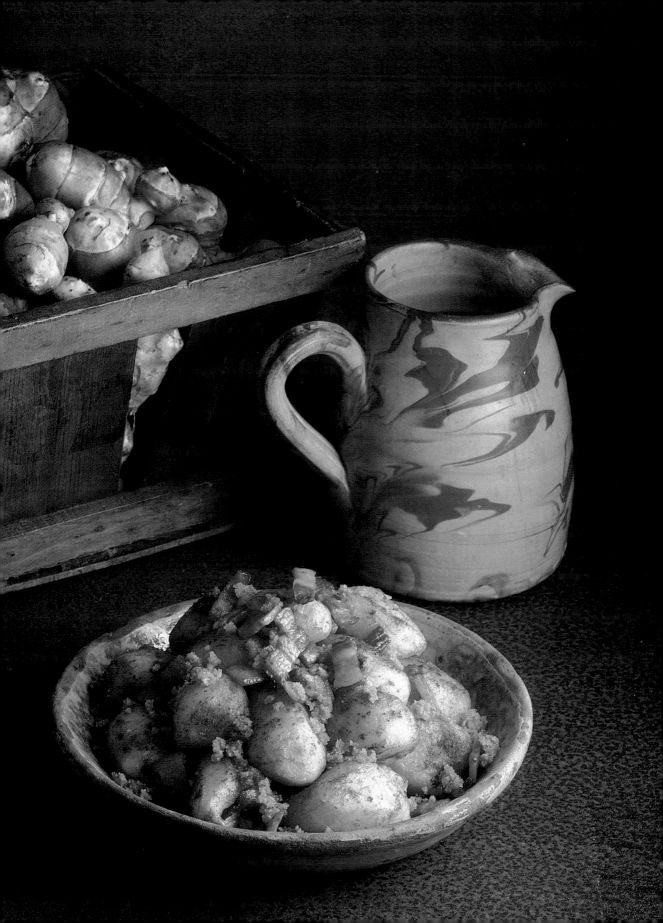

Preparing Jerusalem Artichokes

If you have the choice, pick out Jerusalem artichokes that are as smooth as possible, which will make them easier to peel. Some people eat the skins, but I find them too tough for my taste. I usually just scrub the artichokes then steam or boil in acidulated water in their jackets until tender (or half-cooked depending on the recipe). I leave the peeling until they are done, at which point the skins will pull off easily.

This is not so practical when you want to serve them straight from the pan, embellished with no more than a knob of butter, in which case you'd better peel them before cooking. Their high iron content makes them prone to greying when exposed to the air, so drop them into acidulated water as you peel.

Besides plain cooking, for which they are admirably equipped, they are excellent fried or roasted (parboil first); for soups; mashed with a little potato and plenty of butter to soften the flavour; in stews or in pies with chicken; or thinly sliced and deep-fried to make very more-ish crisps. I've always found that they go particularly well with bacon (maybe grilled to a crisp and sprinkled over a dish of boiled artichokes), and scallops, one of my mother's favourite combinations. Tossed in vinaigrette while hot, and left to cool, they make a fine salad scattered with chopped chives or parsley.

SERVES 4

750 g (1½ lb) Jerusalem artichokes	1 tablespoon olive *or* sunflower oil
Juice of ½ lemon (*optional*)	100 g (4 oz) thickly sliced pancetta *or*
2 teaspoons paprika	streaky bacon, diced
Salt	3 tablespoons fine dry breadcrumbs

Either peel the Jerusalem artichokes before cooking them or vice versa. Steam or simmer them in lightly salted water acidulated with the lemon juice until just cooked but not soft and mushy. Sprinkle the peeled artichokes evenly with a little salt and all the paprika, rolling them around so that they are fairly evenly coated.

Heat the oil in a medium-sized frying-pan. Add the pancetta or bacon and fry over a high heat until crisp and brown. Scoop out with a slotted spoon, letting as much fat as possible drain back into the pan. Drain the pancetta or bacon on kitchen paper.

Add the breadcrumbs to the pan and fry until golden brown. Scoop the breadcrumbs out of the pan, add the hot artichokes and, if necessary, a tiny bit of extra oil. Fry over a high heat for a couple of minutes, turning carefully, until piping hot. Tip into a warm serving dish and scatter with the breadcrumbs and pancetta or bacon.

Stoved Jerusalem Artichokes

This was my mother's favourite way of cooking Jerusalem artichokes, and is one of mine too. I've adapted the recipe slightly from the one she gives in her Vegetable Book *(Michael Joseph), by adding lemon zest to the finely chopped garlic and parsley to make an Italian 'gremolata', one of the best, simple ways to give a lift to practically any savoury dish.*

SERVES 4

1 kg (2¼ lb) Jerusalem artichokes
Juice of ½ lemon
1 tablespoon olive oil
25 g (1 oz) butter
2 tablespoons chopped fresh parsley
1 large clove garlic, peeled and chopped
Finely grated zest of ½ lemon
Salt and freshly grated black pepper

If you are going to save the trimmings for soup, or flavouring a vegetable stock, scrub the artichokes thoroughly. Peel and cut them into halves or quarters if they are large – the pieces should be about the size of a quail's egg or slightly larger, give or take the odd corner. Drop the artichokes into water acidulated with the lemon juice as you work, to prevent browning.

Drain and dry the artichokes. Heat the oil and the butter in a wide frying-pan over a low to moderate heat, until foaming. Tip the artichokes into the fat in a single layer. If you have too many and they are hopelessly heaped up, you'll need to use a second pan, or cook them in batches.

Cover and cook for 10 minutes or so, occasionally shaking the pan gently. Check after 5 minutes and turn them over carefully. After 10 minutes, remove the cover. The artichokes should be beginning to brown. Cook for a further 10 minutes until they are tender, turning occasionally, so that they colour evenly.

While they cook, chop the parsley, garlic and lemon zest together very finely to make a 'gremolata'. When cooked, season the Jerusalem artichokes with salt and pepper and sprinkle over the gremolata.

Chicken with Jerusalem Artichoke Stuffing

A well-flavoured roast chicken – free-range not broiler – with a good stuffing makes a first-class main course for a Sunday lunch. Nuggets of Jerusalem artichoke give this stuffing a most appetizing flavour.

SERVES 4

1 × 1.5–1.75 kg (3–4 lb) chicken
15 g (½ oz) butter
Salt and freshly ground black pepper

For the stuffing

450 g (1 lb) Jerusalem artichokes
25 g (1 oz) butter
2 rashers bacon, diced
1 small onion, finely chopped
1 sprig of fresh thyme
2 tablespoons chopped fresh parsley

75 g (3 oz) soft brown breadcrumbs
3 spring onions, chopped
2 teaspoons chopped fresh tarragon
½ teaspoon Worcestershire sauce
Salt and freshly ground black pepper
1 egg, beaten

First make the stuffing. Boil the artichokes in their skins until just tender, but not soggy. Cool slightly and peel. Chop finely. Melt the butter in a saucepan and add the bacon, onion (not the spring onions), thyme and parsley. Cover and sweat for 10 minutes. Uncover and raise the heat. Cook, stirring occasionally, until virtually all the liquid has evaporated. Cool slightly. Mix with the artichokes, breadcrumbs, spring onions, tarragon, Worcestershire sauce, salt and pepper. Add enough egg to bind.

Pre-heat the oven to gas mark 6, 400°F (200°C). Fill the chicken with the stuffing. Rub the butter into the skin and season with salt and pepper. Roast, basting occasionally, for 1¼–1½ hours until juices run clear. Turn off the heat and let the chicken rest for 10 minutes with the door slightly ajar, before carving.

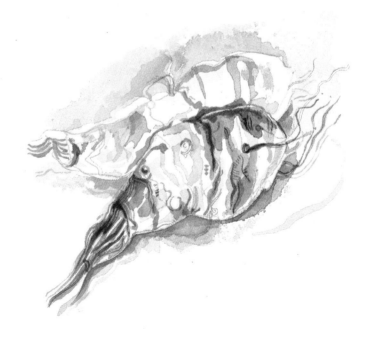

BULBS

Onions • Shallots • Garlic

Leeks

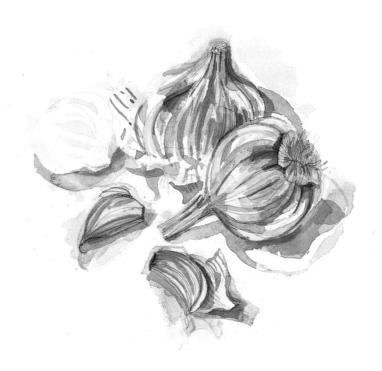

Onions

I had it all straight and shipshape. I knew what was meant by a small onion, an average onion and a large onion. I'd never bothered to stop and weigh them. Why should I? Everyone knows roughly what's what when it comes to onions. But my onion complacency was sorely shaken when I visited the Robinson sisters in Forton just outside Preston. It was a crisp, sunny September day, and when I arrived they were just pulling the last of the year's onion crop. There were still a few rows left waiting, green stems flopping groundwards. Far more than large, these onions were massive.

Susan Redmayne and Margaret Robinson are not just champion onion growers. They are fourth-generation seed merchants, specializing in mammoth strains of onions. So far, the biggest onion they've grown has weighed in at a staggering 3.5 kg (8 lb)!

Size, as we all know, isn't everything. Surely these outsize onions would be pretty tasteless? 'No,' said the sisters, 'absolutely not. We eat them all the time.' And they sent me home with a couple of whoppers, weighing almost 1.5 kg (3 lb) each. Damn it, they were right. The onions tasted as good as any others. The only problem was judging how much of each was equivalent to 'a small onion, an average onion, a large onion' in normal culinary parlance.

In the end I got out the weighing scales and here, for your benefit and mine, is a rough guide to what an onion weighs: small, 75–100 g (3–4 oz); medium or average, about 150–200 g (5–7 oz); large, 225–400 g (8–14 oz). Anything bigger, I now consider to be somewhere from extra large to mammoth.

Whatever their size or colour, onions are good keepers in the right conditions. Leave them somewhere cool with good air-circulation and they'll last for months. Check occasionally and throw out any that are developing soft patches. Don't keep onions in the fridge, especially cut onions, even for short periods of time – unless, that is, you are happy to have onion-flavoured milk and onion-flavoured butter and onion-flavoured anything else that's in there.

Preparing Onions

Right at the opposite end of the scale to the Robinson's onions are the tiny pearl onions, also known as pickling onions, button onions or baby onions. Pearl onions have the dual advantage of being fairly speedily cooked through as well as holding their neat little shapes nicely in long-cooked stews. For casseroles and stews, I usually fry them whole to brown the outside to a good caramel sweetness before adding them to the pan.

They can be fiddly to peel. I swore often enough as I struggled to skin a pound or so of them with a knife, until I discovered a much quicker way to strip them naked. Slice off the root and the tip, then cover the onions with boiling water. Leave for a minute or so, drain, and refresh under the cold tap. Now they should pop satisfyingly out of their tight jackets.

Onions are indispensable in cooking, and that's been true right around the world for thousands of years. In the recipes that follow they are used as a major ingredient, rather than a minor if important flavouring. One of the joys of onions is that they can provide a whole range of flavours depending on how they are used. Raw, they provide a sudden, strong, oniony bite. Cooked fairly briefly until pale and translucent, they soften down to a less insistent mildness. Cooked long and slow they develop a marvellous sweetness. Deep-fried, they are crisp, sweet and savoury all in one. How lucky we are that a vegetable so versatile is also cheap and plentiful enough that we can afford to take it for granted.

Indian Raw Onion Chutney

This uncooked 'chutney' takes only a few minutes to make and is a fine accompaniment to any curry, along with a bowl of mango chutney and sour lime pickles. Try it with the vegetable korma on p. 82. I usually use a red onion which has a sweeter taste than ordinary white ones.

SERVES 4

1 large red onion, finely chopped
1 heaped teaspoon ground cumin
¼–½ teaspoon chilli powder
½ teaspoon sweet paprika
2 tablespoons lemon juice

Mix all the ingredients. Taste and add a little more cumin or chilli if it needs it.

Joyce Molyneux's Onion and Soured Cream Salad

This is so easy and so effective that there's really no need for a recipe proper. Use red or white onions, as you please.

Slice a few onions very thinly. Cover with boiling water, leave for 1 minute, then drain thoroughly and cool. Dress with soured cream, salt, freshly ground black pepper and chopped fresh parsley.

Onions à la Monegasque

Ambrose Heath's The Book of the Onion *was published in 1933. I recently found a copy of the book, packed from cover to cover with recipes that feature onions as an important ingredient, rather than a mere flavouring. This dish is one I particularly like. Small pickling onions are cooked gently in a sweet and sour sauce and served cold. They make a superb addition to a first course, perhaps with cold hams and cheeses.*

SERVES 4

450 g (1 lb) pickling or pearl onions
2 sprigs of fresh parsley
2 sprigs of fresh thyme
1 bay leaf
300 ml (10 fl oz) water
120 ml (4 fl oz) white wine vinegar

3 tablespoons olive oil
3 tablespoons tomato purée
40 g (1½ oz) castor sugar
50 g (2 oz) raisins
Salt and freshly ground black pepper

Top and tail the onions then cover with boiling water. Leave for 1 minute and drain. Slip off the skins and pat dry. Tie the herbs together in a bunch with a piece of string to make a bouquet garni.

Place the onions and bouquet garni in a pan with all the remaining ingredients and bring to a simmer. Simmer very gently for about 1½ hours, until the onions are tender and the sauce is fairly thick. Cool, remove bouquet garni, and serve at room temperature as an hors d'œuvre.

Baked Onions with Goat's Cheese

These baked onions, sweet and tender, filled with goat's cheese and olives, could be served as a side dish to a simple main course, but they are good enough to stand on their own as a first course, or to become an important part of a buffet. They can be eaten hot or cold. I think that they are marginally better hot, but I wouldn't argue the cause too vehemently.

SERVES 4

4 largish onions
100 g (4 oz) young fresh goat's cheese
1 egg
8 black olives, pitted and chopped

½ teaspoon fresh thyme leaves
  or ¼ teaspoon dried
2 tablespoons chopped fresh parsley
Salt and freshly ground black pepper
2 tablespoons olive oil

Peel the onions and cook whole in salted boiling water for 15 minutes. Drain and run under the cold tap. Carefully ease out the centre of the onions, leaving a sturdy shell. Sit the onions shells in an oiled heatproof dish.

Pre-heat the oven to gas mark 6, 400°F (200°C). Chop the onion hearts finely, mix with the goat's cheese, and all the remaining ingredients except the oil. Fill the onion shells with this mixture. Drizzle over the olive oil, and bake for 30 minutes. Eat hot or cold.

Baked Onions with Sun-dried Tomatoes and Rosemary

Totally different in style to the preceding recipe, here the onions are baked in quarters. Choose firm, unblemished onions, of a medium to moderately large size for this dish, but not great big heffalumps. Don't bother peeling them before you begin cooking. The skin comes off very easily after they have been boiled and gives the outer layer a good colour. The sun-dried tomatoes add a welcome sprightly flavour, a fine contrast to the onions.

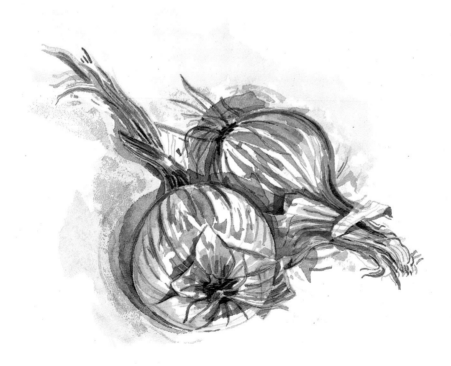

SERVES 4–6

4 onions, unpeeled
6 pieces sun-dried tomato, cut into strips
1 large sprig of fresh rosemary, snapped
    in two *or* 1 teaspoon dried
2 cloves garlic, peeled and chopped

1 tablespoon chopped fresh parsley
Salt and freshly ground black pepper
1 tablespoon white wine vinegar
6 tablespoons olive oil

Pre-heat the oven to gas mark 2, 300°F (150°C).

    Place the onions in a pan and cover with water. Bring up to the boil and simmer for 12 minutes. Drain, peel and quarter. Arrange the quarters in a single layer in a lightly oiled gratin dish and mix in the strips of sun-dried tomato. Tuck the rosemary amongst them, then sprinkle over the garlic, parsley, salt and pepper. Drizzle over the vinegar and then the olive oil. Cover loosely with foil, and bake for 50 minutes. Remove foil, baste the onions with their juices. Continue cooking, uncovered, for a further 20 minutes. Serve hot, warm or cold.

Pissaladière

Pissaladière is made throughout Provence and parts of Northern Italy, but it belongs above all to Nice, where you can buy big squares of it, wrapped in a piece of waxed paper, to eat as you walk through the streets.

    Although it is often made with a bread dough, more like a pizza, I prefer a shortcrust base. The sweetness of the slowly cooked onion and the saltiness of anchovies and olives is set off to perfection by the crumbly texture of the pastry. Some recipes for Pissaladière mix tomato with the onion and good though they are, I think the simpler onion-only topping better. Save the tomatoes to make a salad to serve alongside.

    Pissaladière is perfect for a summer lunch or supper party, or for a picnic. It can be eaten still warm, or cold, as a main course or cut into smaller squares as a starter.

SERVES 6–8 as a main course

350 g (12 oz) shortcrust pastry (see p. 20)
Flour for rolling out

For the filling

3 tablespoons olive oil
1 kg (2 lb) onions, thinly sliced
2 cloves garlic, peeled and finely
    chopped
3 sprigs of fresh thyme
    or ½ teaspoon dried
2 sprigs of fresh rosemary
    or 1 teaspoon dried

1 bay leaf
2 sprigs of fresh parsley
Salt and freshly ground black pepper
50 g (2 oz) black olives (preferably
    Niçoise), pitted
1 tin anchovy fillets, drained and halved
    lengthwise

Roll the pastry out on a lightly floured board to form a rectangle large enough to line a 28 × 30 cm (9 × 12 inch) baking tray. Line the tray with the pastry, prick the base with a fork, then cover and rest in the fridge for 30 minutes to 1 hour while you prepare the filling.

Warm the oil in a saucepan large enough to take all the onions. Add the onions, garlic, herbs and a little salt and pepper. Cover tightly and stew gently over a low heat for 30–40 minutes, stirring occasionally, until the onions are meltingly tender. Discard the herbs. Cool slightly, and add plenty of pepper (no more salt, as the olives and anchovies will ensure that there is no shortage).

Put a baking tray, the same size as the one lined with pastry, in the oven and heat to gas mark 6, 400°F (200°C). Spread the onion thickly on the pastry, arrange the anchovy fillets in a lattice on top and place an olive in the centre of each diamond. Sit the pissaladière on the hot baking tray in the oven (this helps give a crisper base), and bake for 20–25 minutes until browned. Serve cut into squares, hot, warm or cold.

Stir-fried Squid with Onions and Black Beans

This is so delicious, particularly if you can find fresh squid (instead of frozen) which is as tender as butter. The quickly fried onion provides sweetness which contrasts beautifully with the salty black beans. Preparing the squid takes a little time, though it isn't difficult, but once that's done the rest is quick and straightforward.

Salted black beans are available from Chinese food stores, but make sure you are buying the whole beans and not the tins of black bean sauce. Stored in a tightly closed screw-top jar, they will keep for months.

SERVES 4

450 g (1 lb) squid
2 dried red chillies
2 tablespoons Chinese salted black beans
2 tablespoons dry sherry
½ tablespoon sugar
1 teaspoon cornflour
2 tablespoons oil

2 cloves garlic, peeled and chopped
1-cm (½-inch) piece fresh ginger, peeled and finely chopped
2 large red onions, halved and thinly sliced
Salt and freshly ground black pepper

Prepare the squid: pull the head away from the body sac, bringing with it the insides. Discard the head and innards. Chop off the tentacles and reserve. Pull the thin purply black skin off the body sacs. Split sacs open and discard the quill and any gunk left inside. Cut off the 'wings'. Score the inside of the sac and the wings in a criss-cross fashion. Cut the sac into pieces about 2.5 cm (1 inch) across and 5 cm (2 inches) long.

Soak the chillies in warm water for 10 minutes, drain, remove seeds and chop. Mash the black beans roughly with the sherry and sugar, and stir in cornflour.

Heat the oil in a wok (or large frying-pan) over a high heat. When just beginning to smoke, add the garlic, chilli and ginger and stir-fry for a few seconds. Add the red onions and stir-fry for about 2 minutes, until they are patched with brown and softening. Now add the squid and stir-fry for 30 seconds to 1 minute until opaque and curled. Stir the black bean sauce then tip it into the wok. Stir to coat squid and onion and simmer for about 1 minute until the liquid is thickened. Serve immediately.

Pajon
[Korean Spring Onion Pancakes]

One of the many dishes I've enjoyed at my local Korean restaurant is pajon, *a thick 'pancake' of spring onions and other vegetables. It's not a pancake in the European sense, as it is solidly chunky and packed full of bits and pieces. I finally found this recipe for* pajon *in Mark and Kim Millon's book,* The Flavours of Korea *(André Deutsch). Once you've chopped all the vegetables and made the dipping sauce, the cooking is speedy. Serve the pancake as a snack, or in small squares with drinks, passing around the sauce for frequent dunkings.*

SERVES 4–6
For the batter

2 eggs, beaten
225 g (8 oz) flour

1 tablespoon sunflower *or* vegetable oil
200 ml (7 fl oz) water

For the dipping sauce

3 tablespoons rice *or* cider vinegar
225 ml (7½ fl oz) soy sauce
1 heaped teaspoon toasted sesame seeds
1-cm (½-inch) piece fresh ginger,
    peeled, bruised and finely chopped

1 teaspoon ground chilli *or* chilli flakes
1 teaspoon sugar

For the filling

Oil for frying
10 large spring onions *or* 20 small ones,
    split lengthways and cut into 10-cm
    (4-inch) pieces
1 courgette, cut into 10-cm (4-inch)
    matchsticks

1 large carrot, peeled and cut into
    10-cm (4-inch) matchsticks
100 g (4 oz) peeled cooked prawns
Handful of fresh chives, chopped
4 eggs, beaten

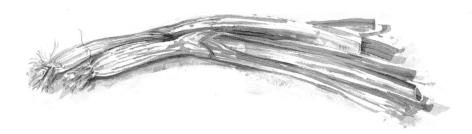

First make the batter: mix the eggs with the flour, oil and enough water to make a medium-thick batter. Let it rest for 15–20 minutes while you prepare the filling ingredients and the dipping sauce. To make the sauce mix all the ingredients.

To make the pancakes coat a large frying-pan with oil and heat. Ladle in a third of the batter. Lay about a third of the spring onions, courgettes, carrots, prawns and chives on the pancakes. Cook for about 5–7 minutes over a medium-hot heat. As the pancake cooks, spoon beaten egg over the filling, to fill in the gaps between the vegetables. When the egg has set and the pancake is well-browned underneath, flip over. Don't worry if it breaks or tears as it will be torn into pieces before eating. Cook for a further 5–7 minutes, pressing down with a spatula to ensure that the batter cooks through.

Remove from the frying-pan, drain on kitchen paper and either serve whole or cut into small squares. Use the remaining ingredients to make another 2 pancakes. Serve with dipping sauce.

Ambrose Heath's Rabbit with Onions

Another recipe from Ambrose Heath's The Book of the Onion *(see p. 92). What is appealing about this recipe is its utter simplicity. You can refine it if you wish, but try it first as it is.*

Next time around, you might want to tart it up – perhaps by flaming the rabbit in brandy before covering or by adding a few quartered mushrooms or chopped tomatoes. Though these are nice additions, they are certainly not essential.

SERVES 4

16 pickling *or* pearl onions	25 g (1 oz) butter
1 bay leaf	1 tablespoon oil
2 sprigs of fresh parsley	1 young rabbit, cut into 8 pieces
2 sprigs of fresh thyme	Salt and freshly ground black pepper

Top and tail the onions and cover with boiling water. Leave for 1 minute. Drain, run under the cold tap, then slip the onions out of their skins. Tie the herbs together with string to make a bouquet garni.

Melt the butter and oil in a heavy, flameproof casserole. Brown the onions in the fat, then scoop out and reserve. Brown the rabbit pieces, then return the onions to the pan along with the bouquet garni, salt and pepper. Cover tightly and reduce heat to low. (If the lid is rather loose, cut a long band of silver foil, scrumple closely round the edge of the casserole, and jam the lid on top.) Stew gently for about 1 hour until the rabbit is tender. Occasionally lift the lid, let the water that has condensed on it drip back into the pan, turn the rabbit, then cover tightly again.

Shallots

S hallots are really a type of onion, but they are a very particular type with their own characteristics that mark them out from the commoner round onion. They grow in tight clusters, joined together loosely at the root. Inevitably, this affects their shape. They may be up to 7.5 cm (3 inches) long, though they are usually a little shorter, but they are squeezed into a slimmer and more elongated form than bulbous onions. There are three main forms of shallot: the 'échalote grise', has a dull grey-brown skin, and a greyish tinge; the 'échalote rose' with its pretty pink flesh; and the yellow-skinned shallot. Some may be pear-shaped, others more elegantly tailored with a gently swelling middle.

Some of the nicest shallots I have ever eaten were grown in Brittany, land of the traditional French Onion Johnny, with his beret, bicycle and strings of onions and, of course, shallots. Having visited sheds where the shallots were spread out on wooden racks to dry for storage, we then sat down to a fine meal based on local produce. With the artichokes there was a shallot vinaigrette (see p. 34), and with the meat there were hot 'Échalotes confites' (see below). The French, quite rightly, appreciate the shallot far more than we do, using it abundantly in cooking. Every year I return from France with big bunches of different types of shallot to hang up in my kitchen.

Échalotes Confites
[Caramelized Shallots]

Like Oded Schwartz's Confiture of Shallots (see p. 100), this is more of a relish than a real vegetable side dish. Unlike the confiture, it is relatively quick to make (and won't keep for more than a few days), and is served hot. It is a lovely accompaniment to roast beef, steak or game, or boiled gammon.

SERVES 4
275 g (10 oz) shallots
50 g (2 oz) butter
1 tablespoon caster sugar
Salt and freshly ground black pepper

Preparing Shallots

The value of the shallot in culinary terms lies predominantly in the flavour – very oniony but with only the mildest hint of tear-inducing pungency. This makes them just perfect for salads or any other raw use. I far prefer small rings of shallot to hefty hoops of onion, scattered over a tomato salad, and I use the shallot vinaigrette (see p. 34) on all kinds of salads. When cooked they have a natural sweetness and gentleness, without being too weedy, that is just the thing for delicate sauces and many other preparations.

There's some value in their size too. Being small, they are handy for one- or two-person cooking, when you might not want to delve into a full-sized onion. They can be pickled, or, far more delicious if you have the time, preserved as a sweet-sharp caramelized 'confiture' (see p. 100). I also use them whole as a vegetable, cooked with butter, stock and sugar, or roast around a joint.

Peel the shallots. If a few are far larger than the rest, take off another layer or two of skin – underneath you will find that they separate into two distinct cloves.

Melt the butter in a heavy saucepan, large enough to take the shallots in a single layer. Fry them for about 5 minutes until patched with brown. Sprinkle with sugar and stir for a minute or so, then add enough water just to cover. Season, stir and bring to a simmer.

Simmer, stirring occasionally, adding more water if needed, until the shallots are very tender and there is only the thinnest layer of syrupy liquid left in the pan. This takes around an hour, but can be done in advance. The cooked shallots keep in the fridge for at least 2 days, and can be re-heated when needed.

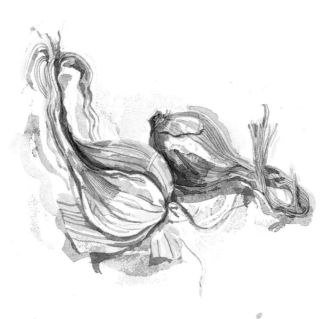

Oded Schwartz's Confiture of Shallots

There is a kind of magic about pickles and confitures which enables them to mellow and mature and take on various characters as they age. Oded Schwartz's Confiture of shallots is fabulous when just made – but if you can resist eating it for a couple of months, or even years, it gets better. Patience is the key to making this sweet-sour confiture. The shallots must be prepared very carefully, simmered quietly over a few days, and left in the cooling liquid overnight, so that they remain intact and take on a lovely, silky, translucent character. In the East, where such confitures originate, this would be eaten as a sweet titbit at the end of a meal, accompanied by a glass of cold water. However, it is wonderful eaten as a relish with cold roast venison, mutton or lamb.

Bird's eye chillies are very small oriental chillies. They are outrageously hot. Use 3–4 larger dried red chillies as an alternative if necessary.

MAKES 2.25 kg (5 lb)

1.5 kg (3 lb) shallots	2–3 small dried bird's eye chillies
200 g (7 oz) salt	2 litres (3½ pints) white vinegar
Water to cover	1 kg (2 lb) preserving *or* granulated sugar
4 cardamom pods	15 g (½ oz) whole cloves
2 sticks of cinnamon	15 g (½ oz) whole caraway seeds
3 strips of lemon zest	15 g (½ oz) ground chilli

Peel the shallots very carefully. It is important to keep the root end as whole as possible, otherwise the shallots will separate during the long cooking. Dissolve the salt in enough water to cover the shallots, and pour over, weighing them down with a large plate. Leave for a full 24 hours.

Tie up the cardamom, cinnamon, lemon zest and the whole chillies in a square of muslin to make a spice bag. Place the vinegar and sugar in a heavy preserving pan or a large heavy saucepan. Add the spice bag and bring to the boil, stirring to dissolve the sugar. Boil steadily for 10 minutes. Skim thoroughly. Add the remaining spices. Drain the shallots and add to the boiling syrup. Reduce the heat and simmer very gently for 15 minutes. Draw off the heat and leave to cool. Cover and leave to marinate overnight.

Next day, bring slowly to the boil, then simmer gently for 15 minutes. Cool and leave overnight as before.

On the third day, bring slowly to the boil again, and simmer very gently, until the shallots are translucent and golden brown. (The high heat of the concentrating syrup caramelizes the shallots.) Bottle in hot sterilized jars (see p. 61), and seal while very hot. Store in a cool, dark place where the confiture will keep for a year or longer, if you can resist eating it, getting more and more delicious all the time.

Stiffado
[Beef and Shallot or Onion Stew]

Though Greek stiffado is usually made with small onions, I like it best made with shallots.
Either way, it is a wonderfully dark, savoury beef stew, perfect for a cold winter's night.

SERVES 6–8

1.5 kg (3 lb) braising beef
1.5 kg (3 lb) small shallots or pickling onions
85–120 ml (3–4 fl oz) olive or sunflower oil
3 cloves garlic, peeled and chopped
150 ml (5 fl oz) red wine
3 tablespoons red wine vinegar
2 bay leaves
1 stick of cinnamon, snapped in two
3 tablespoons tomato purée
Salt and freshly ground black pepper

Cut the meat into large chunks of about 5–7.5 cm (2–3 inches). Slice tops and bottoms off the shallots or onions. Pour boiling water over them, stand for 1 minute, then squeeze out of their skins. Drain well.

Heat half the oil in a large, wide frying-pan and brown the meat, in several batches. Transfer to a flameproof casserole. Brown the onions in the same fat, adding more oil as needed, then add them to the casserole. Pour off excess fat in the frying-pan and add the wine and vinegar. Bring to the boil, scraping in all the brown residue on the base of the pan. Tip over the meat and onions.

Add remaining ingredients and enough water to cover. Bring to the boil, stirring occasionally. Turn down the heat, cover and simmer gently for 2 hours until the meat is tender. Stir it every once in a while.

Uncover and raise the heat slightly. Let it bubble for a further 30 minutes, stirring occasionally. Skim off the fat on the surface. Taste and adjust seasonings. Serve immediately.

OVERLEAF *Stiffado (Beef and Shallot or Onion Stew)*

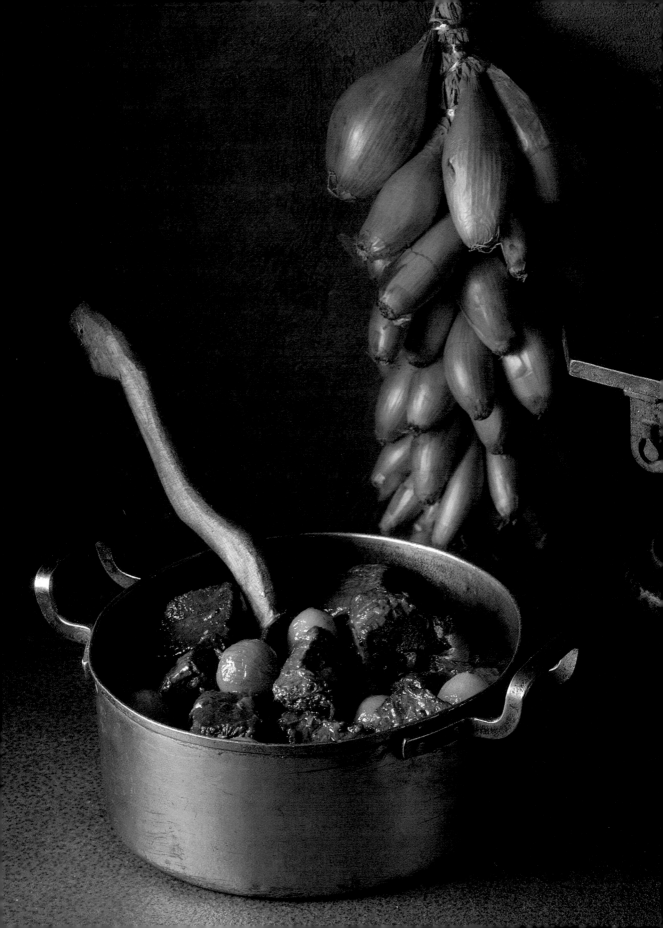

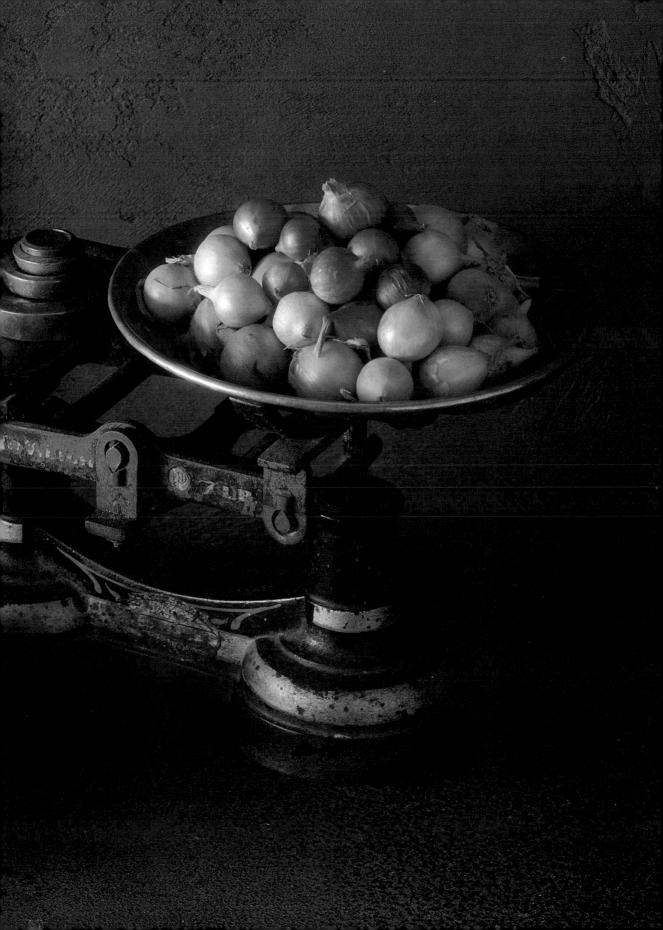

Garlic

Without garlic, we might not have had the great Pyramid of Cheops. Apparently the 300 000 or so slaves threw down their tools and went on strike for an increase in their daily garlic ration. Luckily their demand was granted, the first recorded labour strike was resolved, and the Pyramid was eventually built.

Over the past couple of decades we Brits have learned to love garlic almost as much as the ancient Egyptians did. Sales in the south of the country have even outstripped those of northern France. Some people are still a little unsure about garlic, it's true, but most of the children I meet adore the taste. That's fine by me. I imagine that a good half or more of the recipes in this book contain garlic, chopped, crushed or sliced. Garlic has been so happily accepted, that a couple of garlic cloves thrown into a stew or whatever seems perfectly normal, and garlic bread has become part and parcel of the fast food industry. Even so, some of the recipes that follow in this section may come as a bit of a shock.

I've chosen them because they all use a great deal of garlic – minimum 6 cloves, maximum a hell of a lot more. Yet not a single one of them is so outrageously garlicky in flavour that you will find it hard to swallow. Garlic, cooked in the right way, can become more of a vegetable than an incidental flavouring.

Like onions and shallots, most of the garlic that we buy has been 'cured' or semi-dried. The individual cloves are still juicy (or at least they should be), but enough moisture has been dried off from the outer layers of skin to keep the garlic firm for months on end. There is now a brief season, usualy in late June, for 'green' or 'wet' garlic. These newly pulled, undried heads of garlic have large cloves and are delightfully juicy. Their taste is a little fresher and livelier than cured garlic, but there is not a massive difference. If you do use wet garlic in any of the recipes that follow, you will be surprised to discover that it takes longer to cook than cured garlic. Otherwise, it is totally interchangeable.

Preparing Garlic

The pungency of garlic, fresh or cured, varies from one type to another, the general rule being that the smaller the heads, the stronger they are. The way you prepare it makes a difference too. As the knife slides through the clove it crushes and breaks open the cells that contain the juice. In a few brief seconds a complex chemical reaction takes place and the result is the characteristic smell of garlic. The more finely you chop garlic, the more juice is released and the stronger the flavour. Thinly sliced garlic will be milder than chopped garlic which will be milder than crushed garlic (which can have a slight bitter edge). If you wield your knife thoughtfully, you can control the garlic hit fairly accurately.

With slow cooking, the hot pungency mutes down into soft sweetness, still garlicky, but no longer aggressive. I can't promise that your breath won't smell of garlic after you've eaten, say, an entire roast bulb of garlic bathed in olive oil, but it will have been so delicious that you probably won't care. Cancel the next day's business meeting or romantic tryst if needs be.

Roast Garlic with Herbs

A whole head of garlic per person? Yes, that's right. Whenever I've dished up this first course, my guests have looked horrified at first, but they are soon tucking in gleefully, occasionally complaining that there are no seconds! It has to be eaten with the fingers, so provide plenty of napkins.

SERVES 4

4 heads of garlic
6 tablespoons water
6 tablespoons olive oil

2 sprigs of fresh thyme
2 sprigs of fresh rosemary
Coarse salt

To serve
Rye bread or other good bread, lightly toasted
A handful of fresh herbs (e.g. basil, parsley, chives, chervil), finely chopped (*optional*)

Salt and freshly ground black pepper
2 × 150 g (5 oz) young fresh goat's cheese

OVERLEAF *Roast Garlic with Herbs*

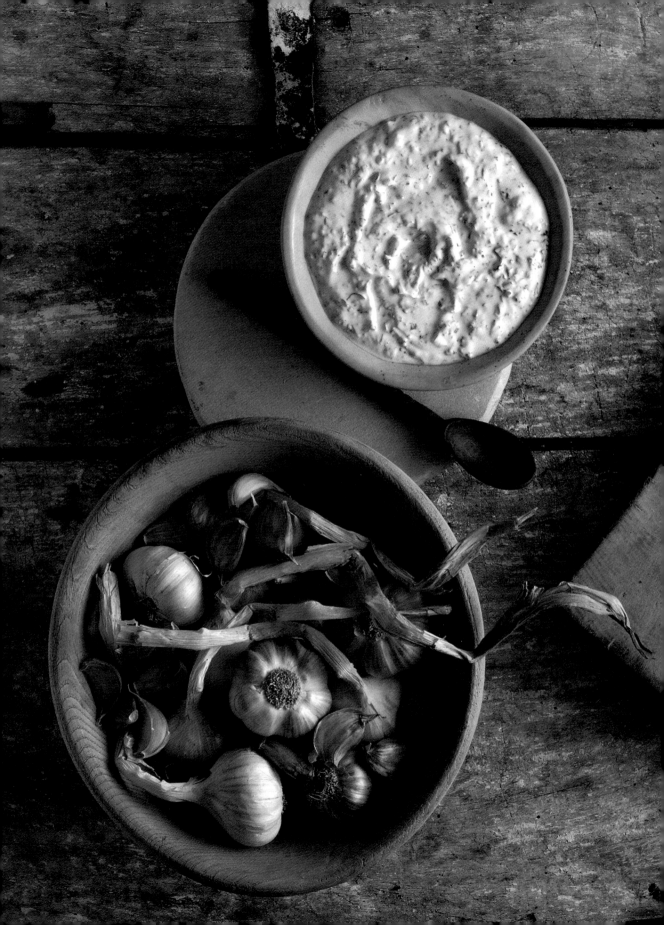

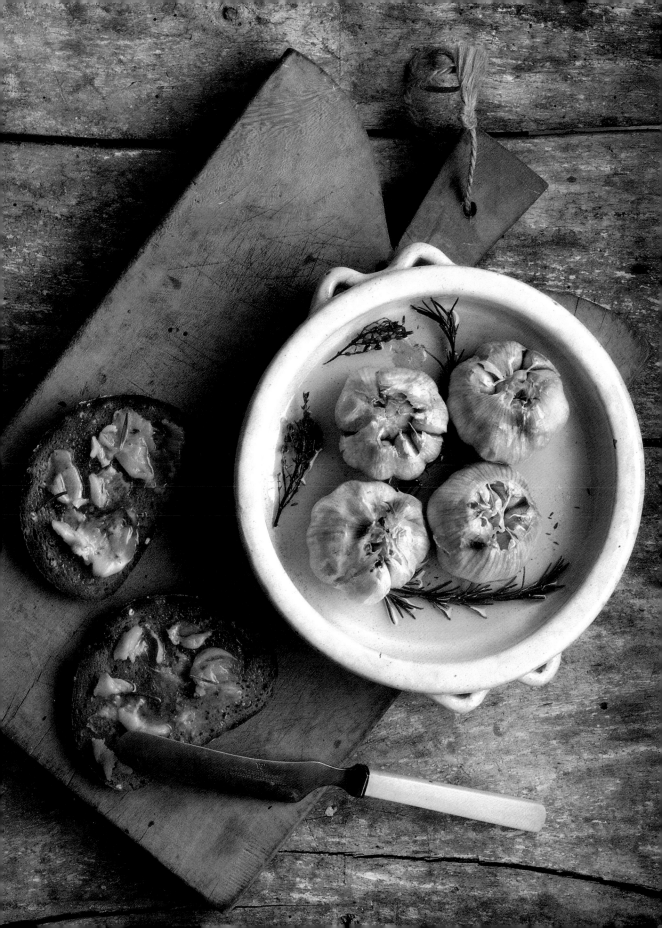

Pre-heat the oven to gas mark 3, 325°F (170°C).

Neaten up the heads of garlic by removing any loose pieces of papery skin. Trim the roots. With a sharp knife cut the papery skin off the top of the garlic, just exposing the very tips of the cloves.

Arrange the garlic heads in a fairly close fitting ovenproof dish and pour the water around them. Drizzle olive oil over garlic heads and tuck the rosemary and thyme around them. Sprinkle with coarse salt. Cover with foil and bake for 30 minutes. Uncover and bake for a further 15–30 minutes, basting occasionally with their own juices, until the garlic is tender and gives when pressed. Add a little extra water if it is drying out.

Beat the goat's cheese with the herbs, salt and pepper to taste, and pile into a bowl. To serve, give everyone their head of garlic and some of the herby cooking oil, slices of toast, napkins and finger-bowls. Using fingers, guests should squeeze the individual creamy cloves of garlic like tubes of toothpaste onto their toast, drizzle with the herby oil, and eat with a dab of soft cheese.

Penny Drinkwater's Provençal Chicken Stuffed with Garlic

Master of Wine Penny Drinkwater is eloquent about every variety and nationality of garlic, but particularly fresh, newly-harvested garlic, as opposed to the semi-dried variety more commonly found in greengrocers and supermarkets. Penny sees garlic not merely as a flavouring but as a substantial and serious element in virtually every dish she cooks – except puddings of course. In her version of Provençal chicken she stuffs the bird with as many cloves as humanly possible, then smears it liberally with butter, before cooking it for up to 4½ hours. This long, long cooking at what seems to be an alarmingly low temperature allows the garlic cloves to soften and caramelize to a melting softness. Surprisingly, the chicken stays moist too.

SERVES 4

4–6 heads of garlic	75 g (3 oz) unsalted butter
1 × 1.5 kg (3–3½-lb) chicken	½ tablespoon chopped fresh tarragon *or*
Salt	fresh thyme leaves

Pre-heat the oven to gas mark 1½, 288°F (145°C).

Separate the cloves of garlic and peel, but leave whole. Season the inside of the chicken with salt and pack in as many cloves as will fit. Smear about half the butter over the opening and the cloves that are peeking out. Season the chicken with more salt and smear the remaining butter over the breast and legs. Place in a roasting tin.

Roast for 3½–4½ hours, basting occasionally with the buttery juices. When the cloves of garlic inside the chicken are very tender, baste the chicken again and sprinkle with the tarragon or thyme. Raise the heat of the oven to gas mark 6, 400°F (200°C) and cook for a final 10–20 minutes, until the chicken is richly browned. Serve hot, with the pan juices, scooping out a generous spoonful of the melting cloves of garlic for each person. Any leftover chicken is excellent cold, with mayonnaise.

Garlic and Onion Purée

I use this purée as a sauce, rather than a vegetable dish, serving it with roast meats, or grilled fish. The slowly cooked onions and garlic develop a marvellous sweetness.

SERVES 6

3 heads of garlic	8 tablespoons olive oil
350 g (12 oz) onions, roughly chopped	Salt

Separate the cloves of garlic, but do not peel. Place in a heavy-based pan with the onion and olive oil. Cover and stew very gently over a low heat until both garlic and onion are meltingly tender – a good 40 minutes or so. Let the mixture cool slightly. Using your hands, squeeze the cooked garlic out of its skins, back into the pan. Liquidize the onions and garlic together, sieve and season. Re-heat when ready to serve.

Broad Bean and Garlic Purée

Grilled garlic gives a soft, smoky garlic flavour – it's strong but not aggressive, highlighting the richness of the purée without being too domineering. Serve the purée as a side-dish-cum-relish or a hot dip.

SERVES 4

450 g (1 lb) shelled broad beans (fresh *or* frozen)	6 large cloves garlic
1 sprig of fresh savory *or* fresh thyme *or* fresh rosemary *or* ¼ teaspoon dried thyme	25 g (1 oz) butter
	6 tablespoons whipping cream
	Squeeze of lemon juice
	Salt and freshly ground black pepper

Blanch the broad beans in boiling salted water for 1 minute. Drain and run under the cold tap. (If they are frozen, just thaw out.) Slip the bright green beanlets out of their grey skins. Finish cooking the beans in lightly salted water with the savory, thyme or rosemary. Drain.

Meanwhile, thread the cloves of garlic on to a skewer and grill fairly close to the heat, until the skin is scorched, and the cloves feel soft. Pull them off the skewer and leave until cool enough to handle. Skin and add to the broad beans. Process or sieve the beans and garlic, put in a saucepan, with the remaining ingredients and re-heat, stirring, until piping hot, smooth and creamy. Serve immediately.

Leeks

The Welsh may brandish leeks as their national symbol, but they can't possibly be any more passionate about their vegetable than the dedicated leek-growers of Northumberland. We're talking serious stuff here – sabotage, sibling rivalry, major prizes, life-long commitment. Morpeth can boast several of the best leek shows of the area, none finer than the one held in the Black Swan pub, always the first show of the year. At least, that's what David Conroy told me, and he's been growing leeks ever since he can remember. He tried to cut back once when his wife decided that she was heartily sick of looking out of her windows over leek-filled polytunnels, but he couldn't bear it. She got her flowers and patio in the end, and he's annexed part of nextdoor's garden to make up for it. Harmony is restored.

All of David's spare time is spent on his leeks and they are, indeed, a magnificent sight. As thick as a weight-lifter's arm, with sweeping long green flags (what you or I would probably call leaves) rising in elegant symmetry from the white base, they are pampered and cosseted throughout their short life.

David's prize-winning leeks may be his pride and joy – when he meets friends for a drink in the Black Swan they talk lovingly about the progress of their 'bairns' – but he's a realist too. The beauty of the big show leeks is purely visual. Though the family may eat one or two when the showing season has drawn to a close, the flavour is comparatively poor and thin. David raises 'pot leeks' of a perfectly normal size for the kitchen.

I like leeks, but I'd always taken them rather for granted. Not entirely unreasonable given that they are cheap and plentiful. They are one of those vegetables that can be quite delicious, but all too often prove a profound disappointment. However, I came home from Morpeth with a healthy new respect for the familiar leek.

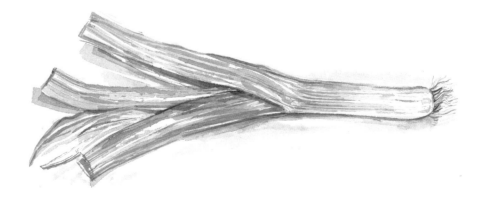

Preparing Leeks

Overboiled leeks are a disaster – slimy and tasteless, they make grim eating. It's even worse when they've not been properly cleaned in the first place. Earth and grit nestle tightly right down inside the layers of leaves, often further in than you might believe possible. They must be thoroughly cleaned before anything else. To do this, trim off most of the flags (the leaves), then slice from the top down the centre of the leek roughly to the middle, or even a little further. A second cut, at right angles to the first, makes them easier to clean, but if you want large pieces you'll have to manage without. Wash the leeks, under the cold tap, splaying them out where you've cut, and making sure you rinse off every last bit of grit.

As long as they are whipped out of the water when they are tender but still with a slight firmness, boiled leeks can be good, but you do have to make sure you drain them thoroughly. I prefer to steam them, so that they absorb less water and retain more flavour. What I like even better is sliced leeks cooked with a little butter or oil in a covered pan over a gentle heat until just tender, or simply stir-fried, perhaps jazzed up with chopped ginger and garlic.

Leeks can also be used instead of onion as a flavouring. Many French fish soups start with sweated leek, and they are indispensable for fish, chicken and vegetable stocks. The coarse green flags need not be wasted either – use them for making soup, or throw them in the stock pot.

Leeks Vinaigrette

Sometimes known as Poor Man's Asparagus, Leeks vinaigrette is a fine dish in its own right. It makes a wonderful first course, served with good bread to mop up the juices. When I can get them, I use slim baby leeks, more like large spring onions, allowing 3–4 per person, but larger leeks work almost as well. Do be careful not to overcook the leeks, and to drain them really thoroughly. Slimy waterlogged leeks are no fun.

SERVES 4

8 medium leeks, trimmed
1 tablespoon white wine vinegar
½ teaspoon Dijon mustard
Salt and freshly ground black pepper
4–5 tablespoons olive oil
1 hard-boiled egg, finely chopped
1 tablespoon chopped fresh parsley

Boil or steam the leeks until just tender. While they are cooking make the vinaigrette: whisk the vinegar with the mustard, salt and pepper. Gradually whisk in the olive oil, a tablespoon at a time. Taste and adjust seasoning. Drain the leeks thoroughly then, while still hot, place in a shallow dish and spoon over the vinaigrette. Leave to cool, then scatter with the chopped egg and parsley.

Coreen Conroy's Leek Pudding

Leek-widow though she may be, Coreen Conroy, wife of Northumberland leek-grower David, does actually like eating leeks. She often makes this traditional leek pudding, varying it from time to time by adding bacon, or scraps of cooked meat. She usually cooks it in a pressure cooker, though I've got to admit that I prefer it steamed in the old-fashioned way but so you can choose your preferred method I've given both with this recipe. When I made it at home, I served it with a tomato sauce – not remotely traditional, but it does add a nice splash of colour and a tartness that sets off the bland suet crust neatly.

SERVES 4

For the suet pastry
225 g (8 oz) self-raising flour
¼ teaspoon salt
75–100 g (3–4 oz) suet

For the filling
4 leeks, chopped
100 g (4 oz) chopped bacon *or* cooked
      meat (*optional*)
Salt and freshly ground black pepper

To make the suet crust, sift the flour with the salt and stir in the suet. Add enough water to make a soft, slightly sticky dough. Knead briefly, dusting with flour to get a smooth, elastic dough. Roll out on a generously floured board to a thickness of about 5 mm (¼ inch).

Blanch the leeks in boiling water for 1 minute. Drain thoroughly.

To cook the pudding in a pressure cooker: line a shallow basin or colander with a large square of silver foil. Line this with the suet pastry, then place the chopped leeks (and bacon or meat, if using) inside and season generously. Lightly flip the pastry over to cover the filling loosely. Don't worry about sealing the pastry tightly – as it cooks it will rise and seal itself. Wrap the pudding loosely with silver foil. Fill the pressure cooker with water to a depth of 5–7.5 cm (2–3 inches), heat and, when hot, stand the pudding inside, cover tightly and cook for 15–20 minutes.

To steam the pudding in the traditional way: tear off a large sheet of silver foil and lay the pastry on top. Place the leeks and bacon, if using, in the centre, and season generously. Flip the pastry over to cover. Enclose loosely in the silver foil, allowing plenty of room for the crust to rise. Boil in a pan of water for 2 hours, topping up with extra hot water as necessary.

Leek and Black Pudding Tart

I find large pieces of black pudding too cloying to enjoy, but cut into smaller pieces and mixed with other things, the flavour is what you notice rather than the texture. I love the combination of black pudding and lots of leeks in this savoury tart.

SERVES 6–8

350 g (12 oz) shortcrust pastry (see p. 20)

For the filling
25 g (1 oz) butter
750 g (1½ lb) leeks, trimmed and thinly
    sliced
150 ml (5 fl oz) single cream
    or half cream
2 eggs
2 tablespoons finely chopped fresh parsley
2 sprigs of fresh marjoram, chopped
    or ¼ teaspoon dried
50 g (2 oz) Gruyère cheese, finely grated
Salt and freshly ground black pepper
225 g (8 oz) black pudding, skinned and
    cut into chunks

Line a 25-cm (10-inch) tart tin with the pastry. Let it rest for 30 minutes in the fridge. Meanwhile place a baking sheet in the oven, and heat to gas mark 6, 400°F (200°C). Prick the pastry base, then line tart tin with foil or greaseproof paper and weigh down with baking beans. Bake for 10 minutes. Remove the beans and paper and return to the oven to dry out for a further 5 minutes.

Melt the butter in a pan and add the leeks. Cover and cook over a moderate heat for 10–15 minutes until tender stirring occasionally. Draw off heat and beat in the cream, and then the eggs, parsley, marjoram and half the Gruyère. Season to taste.

Scatter the black pudding over the base of the tart and spoon the leek mixture evenly over the top. Sprinkle on remaining cheese, and bake at gas mark 5, 375°F (190°C) for 30–35 minutes until just set, and golden brown. Serve hot or cold.

Creamed Leeks with Orange

This cross between a vegetable side dish and a sauce was something I originally came up with to serve with roast pork, and very good partners they were too. However, the creamed leeks are so delicious that I've since served them with all manner of main courses, fish, fowl and vegetable.

SERVES 4–6

5 large leeks, trimmed
40 g (1½ oz) butter
Juice of 1 orange
40 g (1½ oz) plain flour
Salt and freshly ground black pepper
300 ml (10 fl oz) milk
Finely grated zest of 1 orange
Squeeze of lemon juice

Cut the leeks into 4–5 cm (1½–2 inch) lengths then shred finely. Melt the butter in a wide pan and add the leeks. Stir to mix, then add the orange juice and a little salt and pepper. Cover and simmer gently together for 10 minutes or so, stirring occasionally, until the leeks are just tender. Uncover and boil off most of the watery juices until all that remains is a few tablespoons of buttery liquid.

Now sprinkle with the flour and stir to mix evenly. Gradually add the milk, stirring, and then the orange zest. Bring to a simmer and cook for 3–5 minutes until very thick and creamy. If absolutely necessary add a little more milk. Season with salt and pepper and stir in the lemon juice. Taste and adjust seasoning. If not using immediately, spear a small knob of butter on the tip of a knife and rub over the surface to prevent a skin forming. Serve with roast pork, chicken, or fish.

SQUASHES

Courgettes • Marrows

Spaghetti Squash • Squash Flowers

Winter Squashes and Pumpkin

Cucumbers

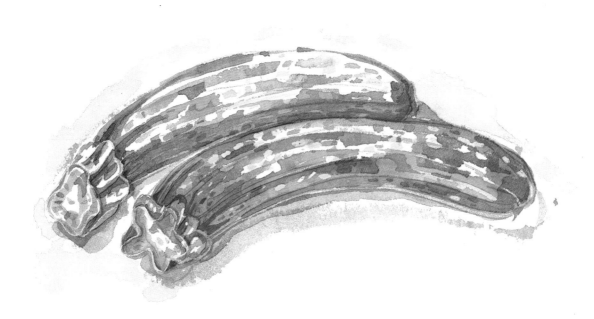

Courgettes

It wasn't easy to find the way up to the fields on the slopes of Solsbury Hill. But what a view when I got there! Out across the sprawling city of Bath, to misty hills and valley beyond.

Henry Whitemore knows the view intimately. He was up here pulling potatoes when the bells rang out on Armistice Day in 1918, a 12-year-old boy at the beginning of his working life. In the 75 years that he's been working these fields he's watched the view change as Bath has grown to cover more and more of the surrounding hills.

Henry's seen the crops grown here change too. There are still a few potatoes and the odd cabbage, but there's more profit in raising bronzed lettuces and courgettes these days. Since the early sixties the demand for courgettes has grown and grown. They're no longer considered exotic as they were just after the war. Henry now works with Tony and Mike Eades, father and 15-year-old son, to supply the local market with all the courgettes they can sell.

The latest change is the addition of sunshine-yellow banana courgettes and an experimental row of new varieties of summer squash. Summer squash is the collective name given to all the plant members of the cucurbita genus that are usually picked young, green and tender-skinned in the summer months. They have pale green to white flesh, and a high moisture content. Their flavour is always mild and gentle. Courgettes are the most familiar of summer squash, but there are others breaking their way into the British scene, such as acorn squashes and the pretty white, yellow or green pattypan squashes.

Gratin of Courgettes with Potatoes and Tomatoes

This gratin looks enchantingly pretty with its closely packed bands of green, red and white, patched with brown in the heat of the oven. As the vegetables cook they will shrink, so it is important to pack them tightly into the baking dish. Overlap them snugly, leaving only about 5 mm (¼ inch) of each slice peeking out. That way, you will get a good balance of tenderness to crispness.

Preparing Courgettes

On the rare occasions when I can lay my hands on really wee courgettes, a couple of inches long and, if I'm lucky, *en fleur* – i.e. complete with flower – I keep the cooking simple, usually steaming, as they are such a treat. Most of the time, I take what I can get, the smaller the better. Big, thick courgettes are best saved for stuffing.

To concentrate the flavour, the first thing to do once courgettes are cut up is to salt them. You've got to allow at least 30 minutes for this to have any effect. A full hour is better. By then a puddle of water will have collected, sucked out from the courgettes by the salt. Wiped clean, some of the salt stays on the courgettes. Rinsed under the cold tap (oddly they don't re-absorb water if you keep it brief) most is removed. Either way, go easy on the salt as you cook – you can always add more at the end.

Boiling sliced courgettes, even steaming them, is a risky business, particularly with large courgettes which have a spongy texture. Leave them a few seconds too long and they'll begin to collapse to a mush. Boiled courgettes are good as a salad (tossed in vinaigrette while hot and left to cool), as long as they are still *al dente*. Otherwise it's a method I avoid. Frying, grilling (my favourite) and baking are what brings out the best in courgettes. Some people like them raw in salads. I don't.

Since little pattypan squashes are so cute, it makes sense to preserve their shape, so keep the cooking simple – steaming whole is your best bet. When they get larger, they are not so good, but can be used as containers. Prepare as for small winter squashes (see p. 131) and bake or steam.

SERVES 4

225 g (8 oz) tomatoes	1 medium-sized red onion
225 g (8 oz) courgettes	½ tablespoon dried oregano
225 g (8 oz) waxy potatoes	3 tablespoons olive oil
Salt and freshly ground black pepper	

Slice the tomatoes and courgettes into discs about 5 mm (¼ inch) thick, then sprinkle them lightly with salt and leave for 30 minutes. Wipe dry. Peel the potatoes, and slice them thinly. Halve the onion lengthways and slice each half thinly.

Pre-heat the oven to gas mark 4, 350°F (180°C). Arrange the vegetables in a single closely

OVERLEAF *Gratin of Courgettes with Potatoes and Tomatoes*

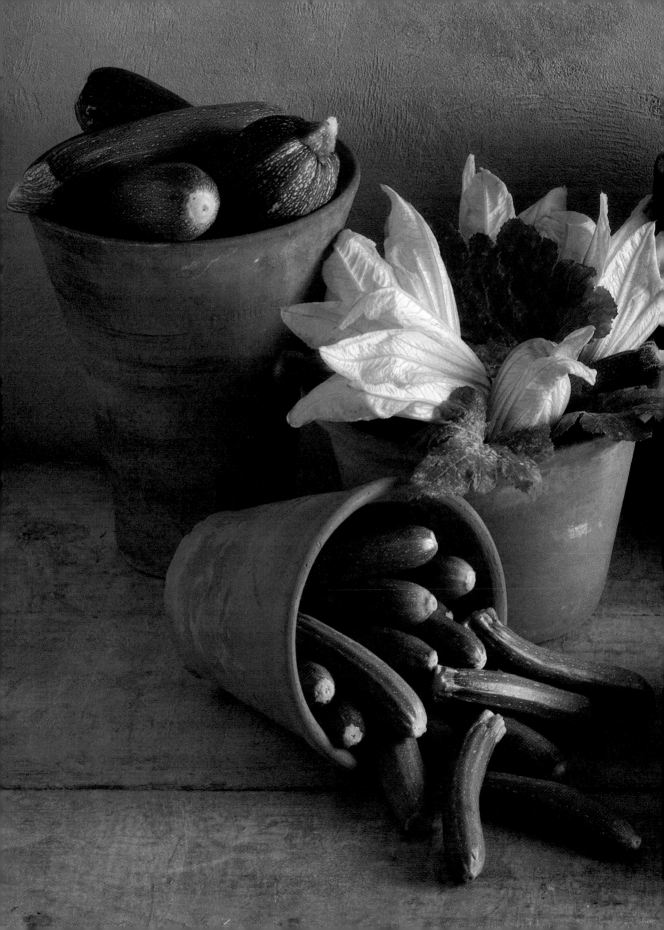

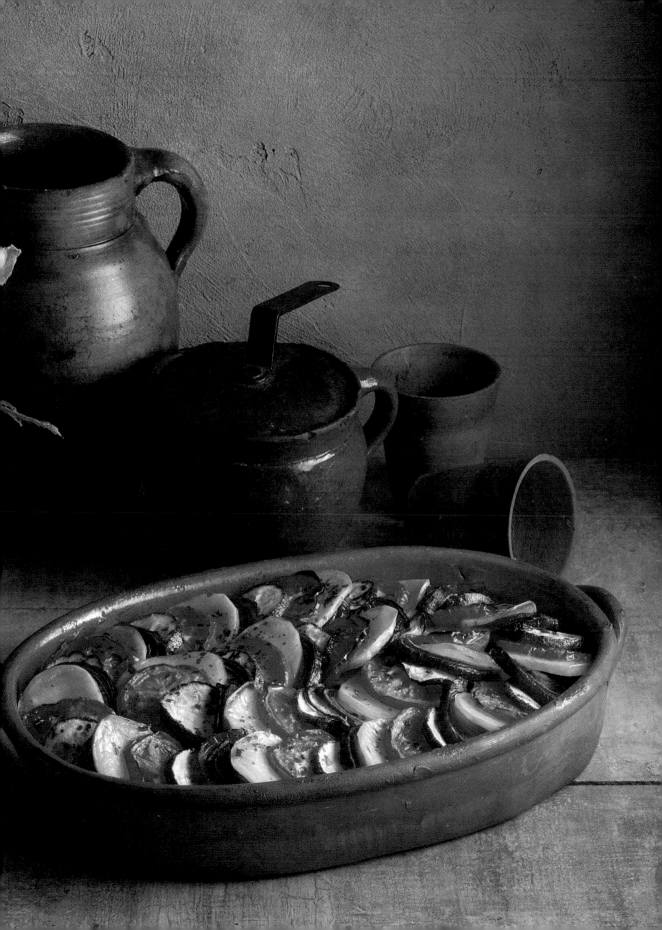

overlapping layer like the tiles on a roof, alternating potato, tomatoes, courgettes and onion, in an oiled heatproof dish. Season lightly with salt but add plenty of pepper. Sprinkle over the oregano. Drizzle over the olive oil.

Bake for about 50–60 minutes, until the potatoes are tender. As the gratin cooks baste 2 or 3 times with its juices, trying not to disturb the arrangement too much. If the gratin threatens to burn cover with foil towards the end of the cooking time. Serve hot.

Wigi's Courgettes in a Bun

Wigi is the cook at rock musician Peter Gabriel's Real World Studios near Bath, where artistes of every race and religion from around the world congregate to record their music. Wigi learned her versatile style of cooking on safari in Africa, watching the locals conjure up meals from whatever was to hand. It's an experience which has stood her in good stead for the unenviable task of cooking supper for everyone from steak-and-kidney-pie-loving guitarists to vegans, often up to 30 of them at a time, and at only an hour or so's notice. She cooks by 'feel', never uses a recipe, and never repeats a dish – but I managed to make a note of this one.

SERVES 4

4 wholemeal *or* white bread buns *or* rolls
50 g (2 oz) butter, softened

450 g (1 lb) small courgettes
Olive oil to serve

For the sauce
2 tablespoons olive oil
5 shallots, sliced, *or* 1 large onion, chopped
2 cloves garlic, peeled and crushed
2 teaspoons turmeric

1½ tablespoons plain flour
600 ml (1 pint) milk
2 bay leaves
Salt and freshly ground black pepper

Cut the tops off the rolls to form lids. Using your fingers pull out the crumb in each roll and lid, to leave a hollow shell. Smear the insides generously with the softened butter. Set aside until needed.

To make the sauce, heat the oil in a saucepan and add the shallots or onion. Stir and cook for a couple of minutes. Add the garlic and turmeric and stir again. Continue cooking over a gentle heat until the shallots or onion are tender, without letting them brown. Add the flour and stir for a few seconds. Gradually stir in the milk. Bring to the boil and add the bay leaves and pepper. Simmer gently until sauce is thick. Season to taste.

Pre-heat the oven to gas mark 4, 350°F (180°C).

Fifteen minutes before serving, put a pan of water on to boil. Put the buns, covered with their lids, in the oven. Re-heat the sauce. If the courgettes are very small and slender, cook them whole, otherwise, quarter lengthwise. Drop the courgettes into the boiling water and cook for 2–3 minutes until just tender. Drain thoroughly. Place the buns on plates and fill with sauce. Arrange the courgettes in the buns, tips hanging out. Drizzle a little olive oil over each, then top with the lid and drizzle over a little more olive oil. Serve immediately.

Grilled Courgette and Pepper Salad with Feta and Mint

The smoky taste of grilled courgettes is very good in salads. Add grilled red peppers and salty Greek feta cheese and you have a salad that is substantial enough to form the main course of a light lunch or can be stretched further to serve as a first course. The courgettes and peppers can be grilled and dressed up to 24 hours in advance, but don't add the feta until you are ready to eat.

SERVES 4–6

450 g (1 lb) small to medium courgettes
Salt and freshly ground black pepper
5 tablespoons extra virgin olive oil
2 tablespoons lemon juice
1–2 cloves garlic, peeled and crushed
   (*optional*)

2 red peppers
2–3 tablespoons roughly chopped fresh
   mint
100 g (4 oz) feta cheese, crumbled

Split the courgettes in half lengthwise. Spread out in a colander, and sprinkle lightly with salt. Leave for 30 minutes to 1 hour to drain. Rinse, and pat dry on kitchen paper. Brush with a little of the olive oil, then grill, turning, until browned and tender. While they are grilling, mix the remaining olive oil with the lemon juice and garlic, if using, and season with pepper and a little salt. Taste and adjust seasoning. As soon as the courgettes are cooked, cut into 2.5-cm (1-inch) lengths and toss in the dressing.

   Quarter the peppers, and remove seeds and white membrane. Grill, skin-side to heat, under a hot grill, until the skin is blackened and blistered. Drop into a plastic bag, knot the ends and leave until cool enough to handle. Strip off the skins and cut into strips. Add to the courgettes, with the mint. Stir, then leave to cool completely.

   To serve, spoon into a dish and scatter with feta cheese.

Zucchine Scapece
[Fried Courgette and Mint Salad]

Another courgette salad, this time from Italy, but it tastes quite different to the preceding one. For Zucchine scapece the courgettes are fried in olive oil and sharpened with red wine vinegar. The smaller the courgettes are, the better they will hold their shape.

SERVES 4

450 g (1 lb) small courgettes
Salt and freshly ground black pepper
3 tablespoons extra virgin olive oil
2 cloves garlic, peeled and sliced

1½ tablespoons red wine vinegar
Small bunch of fresh mint leaves,
   chopped

Trim the ends off the courgettes and cut into 5-cm (2-inch) lengths. If they are thin, cut pieces in half lengthwise. Fatter courgette pieces should be halved then quartered lengthwise. Arrange in a colander, sprinkle with salt, and leave for 30 minutes to 1 hour. Rinse and pat dry on kitchen paper. Fry briskly in the olive oil, with the sliced garlic, until browned and tender.

As soon as the courgettes are cooked tip them into a shallow dish. Add the wine vinegar and mint, seasoning with salt and pepper, turn, then leave to marinate for several hours before serving.

Courgette Omelette

This is a chunky omelette, packed with pieces of tender courgette. The final addition of soured cream or, better still, crème fraîche is entirely optional, but it does make it doubly delicious.

SERVES 2

225 g (8 oz) courgettes
Salt and freshly ground black pepper
5 eggs, beaten
2 tablespoons grated Gruyère cheese
1 tablespoon chopped fresh chives
1 tablespoon chopped fresh parsley

1 tablespoon olive oil
1 large clove garlic, peeled and finely
    chopped
15 g (½ oz) butter
Soured cream *or* crème fraîche to serve
    (*optional*)

Quarter the courgettes lengthwise, then cut into 2.5-cm (1-inch) lengths. Spread out in a colander, sprinkle with salt and leave to drain for 30 minutes. Rinse and pat dry on kitchen paper. Beat the eggs with the Gruyère, herbs, salt and pepper.

Heat the olive oil in a wide frying-pan over a brisk heat. Add the courgettes and sauté until just beginning to brown. Add the garlic and continue frying until browned and tender. Add the butter and stir until it is melted and foaming. Pour in the egg mixture, and cook as for a normal omelette over a moderate heat, pulling up the edges to allow the liquid egg to trickle underneath.

When the omelette is just done – set but still moist on the surface – spoon a couple of large dollops of soured cream or crème fraîche, if using, down the centre, then flip the sides of the omelette over to cover them, and slide out onto a serving dish.

Courgette Risotto

Follow the recipe for Squash risotto, on p. 135, using 450–750 g (1–1½ lb) diced courgettes, and dry white wine. Thyme, marjoram, or rosemary all go well with courgettes, and can be substituted for the sage. If you have courgette flowers, too, stir those in, cut into strips, when the risotto is almost done.

Ratatouille

Like the little girl with the curl, when it's good, ratatouille is very, very good, but when it's bad, it's awful. There are different theories about how to make the perfect ratatouille. Some people insist on cooking all the vegetables separately, combining them only for the last few minutes. True, they keep their individual shapes better that way, but I prefer the other more standard approach. I always cook them together, adding them in stages, so that the flavours all intermingle. The key to making a good ratatouille is, in my opinion, slow lazy burbling on top of the stove (the stew that is, not you or me). Never rush the cooking process. Allow plenty of time for the dish to mellow to a Provençal richness.

There's no point trying to make ratatouille in a smaller quantity than this. And why should you? It keeps well in the fridge for a couple of days, and tastes even better cold than hot.

SERVES 6–8

1 large aubergine	2 cloves garlic, peeled and chopped
450 g (1 lb) courgettes	4 tablespoons olive oil
½ tablespoon salt	1 tablespoon tomato purée
1 green pepper	½ teaspoon sugar
1 red pepper	Salt and freshly ground black pepper
1 × 400 g (14 oz) tin tomatoes	½ teaspoon coriander seeds, crushed
or 450 g (1 lb) fresh tomatoes, skinned	2 tablespoons chopped fresh basil
	or fresh parsley to garnish
1 large onion, chopped	A little more extra virgin olive oil (*optional*)

Cut the aubergine into 2.5-cm (1-inch) chunks. Cut the courgettes into slices about 1 cm (½ inch) thick. Put both into a colander and sprinkle with ½ tablespoon salt. Leave for 30 minutes to drain, then rinse and pat dry on kitchen paper. Halve the peppers and remove stalk, seeds and white inner membrane. Cut into 1-cm (½-inch) wide strips. If using tinned tomatoes, chop roughly in their tin with a sharp knife. If using fresh tomatoes, chop roughly.

In a wide frying-pan, or saucepan, cook the onion and garlic gently in the oil until tender, without browning. Add the aubergine and peppers, stir, then cover and cook for 10 minutes, stirring once or twice. Now add the courgettes, tomatoes, tomato purée, sugar, salt and pepper. Bring to the boil, then lower heat and simmer gently, uncovered, for about 30 minutes, stirring occasionally to prevent burning. Stir in the crushed coriander seeds and continue cooking for another 10 minutes or so until all traces of wateriness have gone and the ratatouille is thick and rich. Taste and adjust seasonings, adding a little more sugar if it is on the sharp side. Serve hot or cold sprinkled with the basil or parsley and maybe a drizzle of extra virgin olive oil.

Marrows

Technically speaking marrows are summer squash but they are the ugly ducklings of the group. Unfortunately, they've already done all their growing up, so will never turn into elegant swans.

Marrow is not a deeply inspiring vegetable. Not unpleasant, either, but it just doesn't set the pulse racing. Even the name sounds dull and heavy. As you will have gathered, I am not a fan. I buy them once in a while, I get given them occasionally, and I've learnt to make the most of them, but I'm not enthusiastic. The key to cooking marrow is to turn its unassuming character into a virtue. Forget plain boiled marrow, or boiled marrow in a white sauce – both culinary disasters. You need to make more effort than that.

Marrow, Potato and Sage Soup

Until recently, I'd considered marrows a waste of time when it came to soup-making. Well, they don't have a great deal of flavour, so it wasn't an entirely unreasonable supposition. I was wrong, as it turns out. Made with a good stock, and fresh herbs, marrow soup can be soothing and most welcome. It's never going to hit the headlines, but when you want something warming and gentle, you could do much, much worse. If you have time, deep-fry a handful of sage leaves for a few seconds, to scatter over the soup just before serving.

SERVES 6

1 onion, chopped
1 clove garlic, peeled and chopped
40 g (1½ oz) butter
750 g (1½ lb) peeled, diced marrow
350 g (12 oz) peeled, diced potato
4 fresh sage leaves
2 teaspoons sugar

1.2 litres (2 pints) vegetable or chicken stock
Salt and freshly ground black pepper
150 ml (5 fl oz) single cream
Chopped fresh parsley or fresh sage leaves to garnish

In a large saucepan cook the onion and garlic gently in the butter until tender, without browning. Add the marrow, potato and sage leaves, turn to coat in the butter, then cover tightly and sweat over a low heat for 10 minutes, stirring occasionally. Now add the sugar, stock, salt and pepper and bring to the boil. Simmer for 20–30 minutes until the vegetables are very tender. Cool slightly, fish out the sage leaves and discard, and then liquidize the soup in several batches. Return to the pan, adding extra stock or water, if necessary. Adjust seasoning.

When ready to serve, bring back to the boil, draw off the heat and stir in the single cream. Garnish with chopped parsley or sage leaves.

Preparing Marrow

As a container for a lively stuffing, marrow is ideal – solid, bland and juicy. There are two ways to stuff a marrow. The first is to cut it into 4-cm (1½-inch) slices and take out the seedy middle, leaving a hole for filling (mound the stuffing up over the marrow, too, so there's plenty with each ring). The second is to cut it in half lengthways and scoop out the flesh to form boats with 2.5-cm (1-inch) thick walls. Either way, blanch the marrow for 4 minutes or so to speed up the baking process. Whatever stuffing you use (ones containing tomatoes and chillies are amongst the best) make sure it is highly seasoned and sprightly, to contrast with the baked marrow. Stuffed marrow will take between 45 minutes and 1 hour to cook in a moderate oven. Cover with foil if it threatens to burn before the marrow is tender.

Stuffing a marrow takes a good deal of time, so unless you have a bottomless pit of marrows to get through, I'd suggest you stick to simpler methods. Cubes of marrow baked with herbs and spices and butter (no water, please) is one of the best quick ways to liven up the vegetable (see below). You might also try simmering it, again cubed, in a well-flavoured tomato sauce.

Buttered Baked Marrow with Aromatics

My favourite way of cooking marrow, without a doubt. Baked with butter, herbs and spices, but absolutely no added water, the marrow's light flavour is preserved at full strength. Vary the herbs and spices as you will (though this seems a particularly appealing combination), but don't tamper with the method!

SERVES 4–6

1 × 1 kg (2 lb) marrow
50 g (2 oz) butter
½ teaspoon dried oregano

1 teaspoon coriander seeds, crushed
1 tablespoon caster sugar
Salt and freshly ground black pepper

Pre-heat the oven to gas mark 3, 325°F (170°C).

Peel the marrow, halve and scoop out seeds, then cut into 2.5-cm (1-inch) chunks. Use about a third of the butter to grease an ovenproof dish that will take the marrow in a tight, single layer.

Spread out the marrow chunks in the dish, sprinkle with oregano, coriander, sugar, salt and pepper, and then dot with the remaining butter. Cover the dish with foil, and bake for 35 minutes. Remove foil, turn the marrow in its own juices, and return to the oven for a final 10–15 minutes until just cooked.

Spaghetti Squash

Vegetable spaghetti, or spaghetti squash, is the most extraordinary vegetable. It looks like a Billy Bunter of a marrow, but it's not until you dig a fork into the cooked flesh that it reveals its bizarre nature. Suddenly the apparently firm pale green interior falls into long slender strands, just like spaghetti. This spaghetti, however, is juicy and slightly crisp. Spaghetti squash is a dieter's dream – very low in calories, which means that a little more cheese or butter might be permitted.

The taste itself is not remarkable, though it is pleasantly fresh. For that reason, it needs generous seasoning and flavouring. The cooked squash can simply be dressed with butter, garlic and freshly grated Parmesan, or it can be given the full treatment with any well-flavoured sauce that you might serve with pasta. One medium squash will feed two generously, or four as a first course, or side dish.

Spaghetti Squash Salad

Most of the time I treat spaghetti squash just like spaghetti, but once in a while I get a creative turn and come up with something a little different. This salad is one example, and probably the best so far. The cooked spaghetti squash is forked into threads, mixed with tomatoes, spring onions and olives and mixed with a sesame seed dressing. Light and fresh tasting, it is lovely for a summer lunch or supper party.

SERVES 6

For the salad
1 medium-sized spaghetti squash
225 g (8 oz) cherry tomatoes *or* firm
    salad tomatoes
6 spring onions, chopped
12 black olives, pitted and roughly
    chopped
8 large fresh basil leaves, roughly torn up

For the dressing
1 tablespoon sesame seeds
2 tablespoons lemon juice
5 tablespoons olive oil
Salt and freshly ground black pepper

Preparing Spaghetti Squash

If you are cooking the squash for a salad, then it can be cut into chunks and boiled for 20 minutes or so, until tender. Scrape the flesh into a sieve or colander and drain well before using.

When you plan to serve the squash in its shell, baking is a better method so that it doesn't become waterlogged. Halve the squash (get a friend to help – it's tough work). Place the halves, cut side down in a roasting tin, and spoon 4 or 5 tablespoons of water around them. Bake, uncovered, at gas mark 4–5, 350°–375°F (180°–190°C) for 30–40 minutes until the skin and flesh can be pierced easily. Drain on a cake rack for a few minutes.

Cook and drain the squash. Make the dressing while the squash cooks. Dry-fry the sesame seeds in a small heavy saucepan over a high heat until they turn a shade darker. Grind to a pasty powder. Mix with the lemon juice and gradually whisk in the olive oil, salt and plenty of pepper. Pour over the hot spaghetti squash and toss. Leave to cool.

Shortly before serving, quarter the cherry tomatoes, or de-seed and dice whole tomatoes. Mix spaghetti squash with the tomatoes and all the remaining ingredients. Taste and adjust seasonings. Serve.

Squash Flowers

One of the pleasures afforded to gardeners who grow courgettes and other types of squash, is an abundance of the egg-yolk yellow flowers. The occasional chi-chi greengrocer may sell them, but they fade and flop quickly, and by the time you get them home they will probably have wilted to a pale shadow of their former selves. To get them at their best, you should pick them in the morning and use within a few hours.

To paraphrase Shirley Conran's famous saying, 'life is too short to stuff a courgette flower'. In my opinion, that's a fiddly task belonging firmly in the domain of the restaurant kitchen. There are plenty of other ways to use the flowers of any of the squash family.

Squash Flower Fritters

A recipe for the lucky few who have ready access to squash flowers. I like to add chopped fresh herbs to the batter, both for colour and flavour, but they are by no means obligatory. The only thing that is obligatory, is that the squash flower fritters should be eaten as soon as they come out of the pan, while they are still hot and crisp. Gather family and friends together in the kitchen with you and hand them round as soon as they are done, but make sure you get your fair share.

SERVES 4

12–16 squash flowers
Lemon wedges
Oil for deep-frying

For the batter
100 g (4 oz) plain flour
Salt and freshly ground black pepper
2 eggs, separated
2 tablespoons olive oil
3 tablespoons dry white wine
2 tablespoons finely chopped fresh herbs
    (e.g. parsley, basil, chives, chervil),
    (*optional*)

Preparing Squash Flowers

My favourite way to eat them is encased in a crisp coating of light batter and for that I give a recipe overleaf. If you have only a few flowers, use them as a garnish: deep-fry the petals briefly without batter or any other coating and they will crisp to a remarkable translucent gold. You don't have to cook them at all, though. Squash flowers have a sweet, nutty flavour when eaten raw and make a pretty addition to any summer salad, or can be shredded and scattered over soups or a courgette risotto (see p. 122) just before serving.

To make the batter, sift the flour into a bowl and add salt and pepper to it. Make a well in the centre and add the egg yolks, olive oil and wine. Stir, gradually drawing in the flour and adding enough water to make a batter with the consistency of thickish single cream. Stir in the herbs, if using. Rest the batter for 30 minutes. Just before using, whisk the egg whites stiffly and fold into the batter. Dip the flowers into the batter, holding them by their stems, then deep-fry until puffed and golden. Serve immediately with lemon wedges.

Winter Squashes and Pumpkin

Ralph and Barbara Upton grow and sell over 60 different varieties of squash or 'cucurbita'. Drive down the road towards their cottage in the Sussex village of Slindon in the early autumn and your eye is suddenly caught by myriad splashes of orange, yellow, white and silvery-blue. Draw closer and the shapes materialize into hundreds of squashes and pumpkins – spotted, striped, knobbly, smooth, big and little, hanging from the rafters, congregating in the yard on bales of hay, tumbled into wheelbarrows, piled high on the rooves of the sheds, and heaped up inside. It's the most unlikely and beautiful sight in this peaceful corner of Sussex.

In their quiet way, the Uptons have pioneered the squash in this country. Supermarkets now sell a few varieties in the autumn – usually butternut, turban squash, pumpkin and occasionally acorn squash. Good wholefood shops will have a greater choice and West Indian food stores may sell a Caribbean variety.

The American term 'winter squash' covers all of those members of the cucurbita group which have tough, hard rinds and keep for at least a month or two, often much longer. With a few exceptions, the flesh is yellow to orange. Pumpkins are a type of winter squash, though again, there are several varieties. What marks them out is their tremendous size. The Uptons' record breaking pumpkin weighed in at over 27 kg (60 lb).

The same name may be used for several different types of squash, and one variety may be known by a whole host of names. It can all get quite confusing but don't let this put you off. For most purposes, one type of squash is as good as another. Of course, you'll get slightly different results from each and you may have to adapt recipes slightly, but that's part of the fun.

Winter squashes can be stored until needed in a cool airy place – a dry garage is ideal – but once you've cut into a squash, use it straight away, even if that means cooking and freezing what you can't eat immediately.

Preparing Winter Squashes

Baking is by far the best method for cooking squashes. Don't boil them, unless the liquid is to be used as part of the finished dish, e.g. when making a soup. Too much of their flavour seeps out into the water, leaving behind nothing but a tasteless water-logged mass of orange. The only exceptions to this rule are the smaller squashes which can be boiled whole and, at a pinch, the spaghetti squash (see p. 127).

The more densely fleshed squashes, such as butternut or the New Zealand Crown Prince, can be cut into large cubes and roasted round a joint like potatoes or parsnips.

To bake a large wedge of pumpkin or other squash, remove the seeds but not the skin, wrap it in oiled or buttered foil and bake at any temperature between gas mark 3–6, 325°–400°F (170°–200°C) until tender. Serve it plain, or mashed with plenty of butter and/or cream, salt, pepper and spice. Or purée and drain it for use in pies (see p. 132), cakes, and breads.

To cook small squashes, such as Little Dumpling, cut off the tops to form lids, then, using a sturdy spoon, a small knife and/or your fingers, pull out the fibres and seeds. Insert a knob of butter and salt and pepper (or for a fancier finale add chopped herbs, lemon zest and perhaps some single cream), replace the lid and stand in a baking dish, surrounded by a few tablespoons of water. Bake at gas mark 4–5, 350°–375°F (180°–190°C) until tender. Check occasionally adding a little more water if the squashes are dry. Cover with foil if they threaten to burn – though they shouldn't as they will be done within half an hour. Test by lifting a lid and prodding the inside. Serve as they are, or use as containers for little stews and ragouts. Acorn squashes with their pointy ends are often classified as summer squashes, but cooked like winter squashes. Cut them in half lengthways, remove the seeds, then bake in halves with butter, protected by foil.

To make a container from a larger squash or pumpkin, cut off a lid, remove seeds and fibres, smear butter liberally over the inside and season. Replace the lid and wrap in foil. Stand in a baking dish or oven-proof bowl that will support the sides of the squash. Bake more slowly at gas mark 3–4, 325°–350°F (170°–180°C) erring marginally on the side of undercooking, so that the squash doesn't collapse the moment you fill it up.

Preparing Pumpkin or Squash Purée

Take a 1.25 kg (2½ lb) wedge of pumpkin or other winter squash, or 3 large butternut squashes. Cut in half if necessary, and remove seeds and fibres in the centre. Set the pumpkin or squashes on an oiled baking tray, cut sides down, cover with foil and bake at gas mark 5, 375°F (190°C) until soft – anything from 40 minutes to 2½ hours! Leave on the trays until cool enough to handle. Scoop out the pulp and process until smooth, or pass through the fine blade of a mouli-légumes. Tip into a colander lined with split-open coffee filters or a double layer of muslin and leave to drain overnight. Weigh out amount required. Any leftover pulp can be frozen.

Frances Bendixon's Ultimate Pumpkin Pie

There are as many recipes for pumpkin pie (the essential American Thanksgiving dessert) as there are people who make it. Although Frances Bendixon's ancestors were members of the Plymouth Brethren who set sail for New England on the Mayflower *back in the seventeenth century, she makes no claims to cooking the authentic pumpkin pie. She cooks the* ultimate *pumpkin pie. The secret is to use double cream (rather than milk or evaporated milk) and, most importantly, to drain the pumpkin purée overnight. This long draining to eliminate any wateriness makes all the difference between a take-it-or-leave-it pumpkin pie, and a very more-ish one. It's a trick worth remembering when making other recipes which require pumpkin purée. Frances Bendixon's pumpkin pie is so rich that it really doesn't need any embellishment. However, if you insist on going right over the top, serve it with whipped cream flavoured with brandy, or a scoop of vanilla ice-cream.*

SERVES 6–8

275 g (10 oz) shortcrust pastry (see p. 20)

For the filling
2 large eggs (size 1 or 2)
400 g (14 oz) thoroughly drained
    pumpkin *or* squash purée (see above)
1½ teaspoons ground cinnamon
½ teaspoon ground ginger
½ teaspoon ground allspice
½ teaspoon salt
250 ml (8 fl oz) double cream
120 ml (4 fl oz) maple syrup *or* to taste

Place a baking sheet in the oven and heat to gas mark 7, 425 °F (220 °C). Line a deep 23-cm (9-inch) pie plate or tart tin with the pastry. Use a fork to decorate the rim. Prick the base with a fork. Chill until needed.

Beat the eggs, then beat in the pumpkin or squash purée, followed by the spices and salt and then the cream. Add the maple syrup gradually, tasting as you do so. If you used a sweet squash then you may not need all of it. Taste and add extra spices if you think it needs a little more pepping up. Pour the mixture into the prepared pastry case.

Place the filled case on the hot baking sheet in the oven. Bake for 10 minutes to start the crust browning, then reduce heat to gas mark 5, 375°F (190°C) and cook for about another 30 minutes or until the filling looks set around the edges and about halfway to the middle of the pie, but the centre is still a bit wobbly. Serve warm or cold.

Chinese Scrambled Egg with Squash

When Frances Bendixon was buying the pumpkin for her pumpkin pie (see opposite) her Chinese grocer told her how she liked to cook winter squash with eggs. Frances didn't get round to trying it, but she passed the idea on to me. It turns out to be an excellent, if unusual, way to turn squash into a light main course.

SERVES 2

175–225 g (6–8 oz) piece of pumpkin *or* other winter squash (e.g. butternut)
4 eggs
Salt and freshly ground black pepper

2 tablespoons oil
1 clove garlic, peeled and chopped
1-cm (½-inch) piece of fresh ginger, peeled and finely chopped

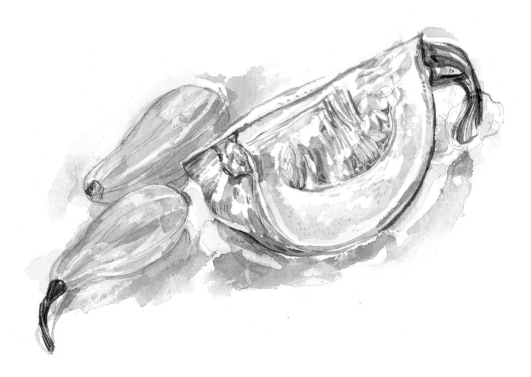

Cut off the rind and remove seeds and fibres from the pumpkin or squash. You should end up with around 100 g (4 oz) of flesh. Slice very thinly, then cut the slices into narrow batons, about 2.5–4 cm (1–1½ inches) long. Beat the eggs, adding salt and pepper.

Heat the oil in a wok over a high heat until hazy. Add the garlic and ginger and stir-fry for a few seconds. Add the squash and stir-fry until lightly browned and tender. Pour in the beaten egg and quickly stir and scramble until beginning to set. Scoop into a dish and serve.

Pumpkin Soup in a Pumpkin

I've always liked soup with plenty of bits and bobs in it, and this one has its fair share. Once you've prepared the pumpkin, all there is to do is fill it up and pop it into the oven to get on with the cooking all by itself. Exact cooking time depends on the size of the pumpkin, but if it seems to be almost done and you are not yet ready to eat, turn the oven down low to prevent the shell softening too much.

SERVES 4

1 × 1.75–2.25 kg (4–5 lb) pumpkin
15 g (½ oz) butter
Salt and freshly ground black pepper
50 g (2 oz) long-grained rice
2 shallots, finely chopped
2 cloves garlic, peeled and finely chopped
600–900 ml (1–1½ pints) milk

2 sprigs of fresh thyme
1 sprig of fresh rosemary
1 tablespoon finely chopped fresh parsley
25 g (1 oz) freshly grated Parmesan cheese
Crisp croûtons to serve

Pre-heat the oven to gas mark 4, 350°F (180°C).

Using a sharp knife, cut a lid off the pumpkin. Scrape out the seeds and threads inside and discard. Rub the butter around the inside of the pumpkin and season generously with salt and pepper. Place rice, shallots, and garlic in the pumpkin. Add the thyme, rosemary, and parsley. Bring the milk to the boil, and pour enough into the pumpkin to almost fill it. Cover with its lid, then wrap foil loosely around it, taking care not to spill the contents. Stand in a roasting tin and bake for 1¾–2½ hours until the inside is tender.

If you can find them, fish out the herb twigs, then stir the Parmesan into the soup, taste and adjust the seasoning. As you serve the soup, scrape out some of the softened pumpkin with each spoonful. Pass croûtons around separately.

Squash Risotto

I've made this risotto with several different types of squash, all of them good, but the sweet dumpling (also known as little apple) squash has come out top of the league. It has a pretty cream-coloured skin streaked with green, and a firm texture and sweet taste. Try it if you find it.

The final addition of cheese is optional. With a sweet dumpling, I found it unnecessary, but with other less sugary squashes it adds a final lift. Taste the risotto before you add it and see what you think.

SERVES 4–6

1 × 750 g (1½ lb) winter squash
   or a wedge of pumpkin
1 onion, chopped
75 g (3 oz) butter
1.2 litres (2 pints) chicken *or* vegetable
   stock
4 fresh sage leaves, torn up
350 g (12 oz) Arborio rice

2 medium-sized tomatoes, skinned,
   de-seeded and chopped
1 large glass dry white wine
Freshly ground black pepper
2 tablespoons chopped fresh parsley
2½ tablespoons freshly grated Parmesan
   cheese (*optional*)
Extra freshly grated Parmesan cheese to
   serve (*optional*)

Cut the squash into 1-cm (½-inch) cubes, discarding skin and seeds. In a heavy-based saucepan, large enough to take all the ingredients with room to spare, cook the onion in half the butter until tender, without browning. Meanwhile bring the stock to the boil in a separate pan. Turn the heat down as low as possible to keep hot, without actually boiling.

Add the sage and pumpkin to the onion and stir for about a minute, before adding the rice. Continue stirring for another minute. Now add the tomatoes, wine, salt and pepper, and simmer, stirring, until the wine has evaporated. Add a couple of ladlefuls of the hot stock. Simmer, stirring, until the liquid has evaporated. Repeat until the rice is tender but still *al dente*. Stir in the remaining butter, parsley, Parmesan (if using) and more pepper and salt if needed. Let it sit for a minute or so, then serve with more Parmesan to hand round if you like.

Squash and Aubergine Risotto

Follow the recipe for Squash Risotto (above) but replace 250 g (8 oz) of the squash with 1 large aubergine, cut into ½-inch cubes, without peeling. Add the aubergine at the same time as the squash.

OVERLEAF *Squash and Aubergine Risotto*

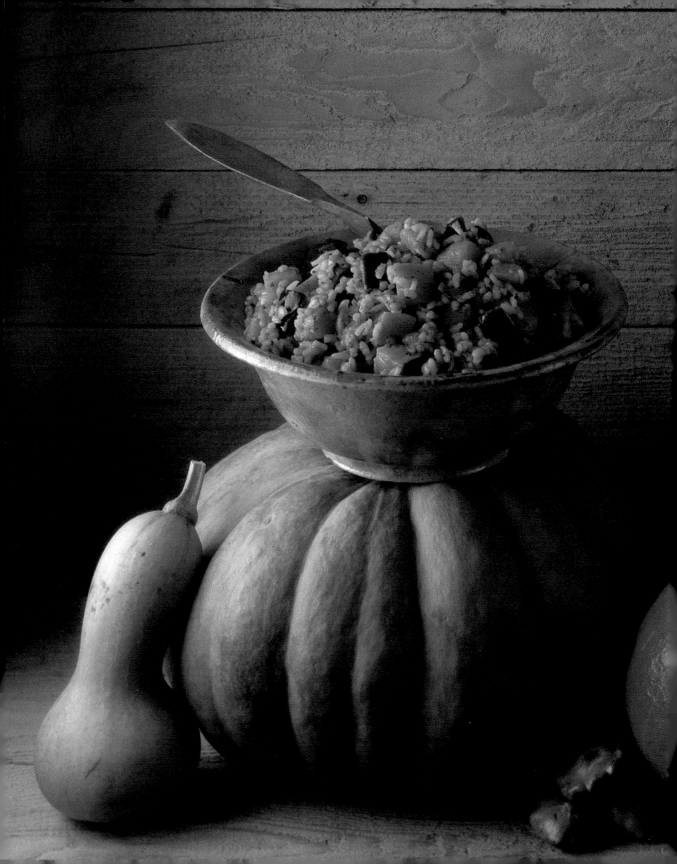

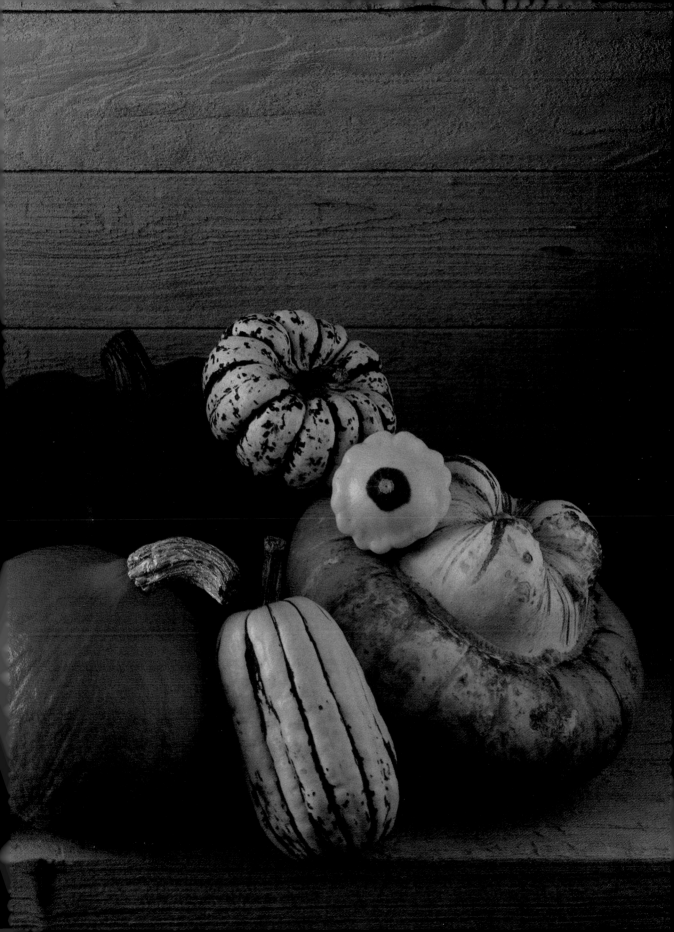

Turkish Candied Squash

A friend of the family gave a recipe for this Turkish pudding to my mother many years ago. It quickly became a family favourite. Since then, I've come across it in Turkish cookery books with slight variations, but always the same basic intent. It is the best pumpkin or squash pudding I have ever come across, but it is very sweet indeed, so serve in small portions.

A fairly densely fleshed squash, such as butternut or Red Kuri is easiest to handle. Straight pumpkin is softer and has a tendency to collapse, but as long as you don't mind the pudding looking a little mushier than it should, pumpkin does a fine job.

SERVES 4–6
1-kg (2-lb) wedge of winter squash (e.g.
　　Red Kuri *or* butternut *or* pumpkin)
225 g (8 oz) caster sugar
120 ml (4 fl oz) water

To serve
Crème fraîche, whipped cream *or* Greek
　　yoghurt
100 g (4 oz) walnuts, roughly chopped

Trim off the rind and discard the seeds of the squash, then cut into 2.5-cm (1-inch) chunks. Layer with the sugar in a wide saucepan and pour over the water. Cover tightly, and cook over a very low heat for about 1 hour, turning the pumpkin carefully occasionally. Towards the end of the cooking time have a look in the pan to assess the liquid level. If it is copious, uncover and let the liquid boil down to a thick syrup. Cool in the pan.

Spoon into individual dishes and chill.

To serve, top with a dollop of crème fraîche, cream or yoghurt, then scatter with walnuts.

Indian Spiced Squash

In theory, this exotically buttery spiced mash of pumpkin or squash should be enough to feed four, but I'll admit to greedily downing more than my quarter share on several occasions. It is hopelessly more-ish.

This recipe is one exception to the rule that pumpkin and squash should not be cooked in water. The liquid becomes an integral part of the spiced purée, so no flavour is lost. If there still seems to be a copious lake of liquid when the pumpkin is done, boil hard for a few minutes to reduce.

Star anise is a spice with a superb aniseed flavour, much used in oriental cooking and now very fashionable in smart restaurants. Buy it from good delicatessens or oriental food stores.

Serves 4

1–1.25 kg (2–2½ lb) wedge of pumpkin
    or orange winter squash
      (e.g. butternut)
½ star anise
¼ teaspoon turmeric
1 bay leaf
1 teaspoon sugar
Salt
50 g (2 oz) lightly salted butter
2 tablespoons oil
1 small onion, chopped

½ tablespoon cumin seeds, coarsely
    crushed
½ tablespoon coriander seeds, coarsely
    crushed
2 cloves garlic, peeled and chopped
2.5-cm (1-inch) piece fresh ginger,
    peeled and grated
1–2 green chillies, de-seeded and
    chopped
Handful of fresh coriander leaves

Peel the pumpkin, discard the seeds, and cut into 2.5-cm (1-inch) chunks. Place in a saucepan with the star anise, turmeric, bay leaf, sugar and salt. Add 150 ml (5 fl oz) water, bring to the boil, then cover and simmer gently, stirring occasionally until the pumpkin is very tender – about 20 minutes. Do not drain.

Just before serving, re-heat the pumpkin. Heat the butter with the oil in a small saucepan over a fairly high heat. Add the onion, and fry until golden. Raise the heat and add the crushed cumin and coriander seeds, frizzle for about 20 seconds, then add the garlic, ginger and chilli and cook for about a minute more. Transfer the pumpkin to a warm serving dish, mashing it slightly as you do so, and pour over the sizzling butter. Stir lightly to streak the butter into pumpkin, then scatter with coriander leaves and serve.

Mrs Upton's Pumpkin Marmalade

Surrounded as she is every autumn with her husband's spectacular squashes and pumpkins (see p. 130), it's not surprising that Barbara Upton has gathered together a wealth of recipes over the years. This pumpkin marmalade is a relatively new member of the collection but has fast established itself as a firm favourite. Though it is called a marmalade it won't actually gel in the usual way. The thing is to cook the mixture long enough for the syrup to thicken and reduce down. That way it will be jammy enough to spread on toast, even if it isn't technically a real jam.

Makes about 1.75 kg (4 lb)

1 kg (2 lb) pumpkin *or* other winter
    squash (weighed after removing skin
    and seeds)

1 kg (2 lb) granulated sugar
2 oranges
250 ml (8 fl oz) water

Cut the pumpkin or squash into small cubes. Mix with the sugar in a large bowl. Slice the oranges thinly and cut the slices roughly into quarters. In a separate bowl cover with the water. Leave both bowls to stand for 24 hours, stirring the pumpkin occasionally.

Put the oranges and water in a large saucepan and bring to the boil. Add the pumpkin and sugar and bring gently to the boil, stirring to dissolve the sugar. Boil until the mixture is thick and syrupy – about 30 minutes. Pour into sterilized jars (see p. 61) and seal.

Cucumbers

Cucumbers are not, botanically speaking, squashes proper, but they are closely realted, and like their cousins, they can be trained to climb up strings and poles. My first taste of a freshly picked cucumber was a moment of revelation. Until then I'd liked cucumbers well enough – juicy, cool and refreshing green torpedos that made great sandwiches – but I would never have ascribed any depth of flavour to them. This one was different. It was sweeter than a bought cucumber, with a pronounced cucumbery taste. My first thought? That it would make the ultimate cucumber sandwich . . . was there any bread and butter to hand?

We'd pulled the cucumber in question off a plant in potter Janet Allan's vegetable potager, and sliced it right there on the spot. Ever since she tasted her first home-grown cucumber, Janet has been unable to bring herself to buy them, and there are cucumber plants enough in the garden to keep her amply supplied right through the summer.

She's even trained one cucumber vine to twist up and over the long willow arch that leads into the potager. By the end of the summer, she was hoping to be able to pluck cucumbers from its curves as she wanders through to tend the rest of the vegetables. In the meantime the vine is entangling itself amongst scarlet runners, purple French beans, squashes, and yellow-flowered canary creeper – a riot of greenery splashed with brightly coloured flowers creating a shady passage from the pleasure garden to the practical potager.

Back at home, I had to return sadly to the plastic-clad cucumbers of the supermarkets. I made myself a cucumber sandwich and that cheered me up no end. As long as cucumbers are firm from one tip right through to the other, they are good enough to provide pleasure even if they don't quite measure up to a freshly picked cucumber.

Preparing Cucumbers

Don't imagine that cucumbers are only good for sandwiches and salads, fine institutions though both can be. There's greater potential in a cucumber than that. It's not often that we think of cooking cucumbers and yet why not? Wedges of cucumber, simmered until just tender, then well drained and finished in a little butter, or glazed with sugar and butter are surprisingly delicious. Or they can be sliced in half, scooped out to form boats and filled with a well-seasoned stuffing to be baked in the oven.

In a covered pan, stew cucumber wedges or 'olives' gently in butter with salt and pepper, until tender. Serve them up with fried fillets of sole, brill or whiting, and you have the classic Poisson Doria. Cook them in just the same way and finish by simmering in cream for a few minutes and sharpening with a squeeze or two of lemon juice to make a much richer cucumber sauce that goes well with fish or chicken.

Whether I'm using cucumbers raw or cooked, I rarely bother to peel them. I like the look of dark green against pale. I make an exception only for the paper-thin salad on p. 142 and sometimes for the delicious pickles on p. 143. Some people find the skins indigestible, and if you're one of them you will peel the skins off whatever I say. Never bother removing the seeds unless you intend to stuff the cucumbers. Otherwise it is a totally pointless exercise. I suppose if the cucumber was enormous and the seeds beginning to toughen it might be necessary, but I've never yet come across a cucumber that old and past it.

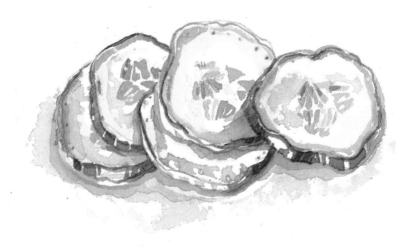

Tzatziki Soupa
[Chilled Yoghurt and Cucumber Soup]

This soup demands precious little effort and no cooking whatsoever. What more could you ask for on a hot summer's day? Present it well chilled with a flourish of fresh mint and you have a first course fit for kings.

SERVES 6

1 cucumber
600 ml (1 pint) Greek-style yoghurt
1–2 cloves garlic, peeled and crushed
Finely grated zest of 1 lemon

2 tablespoons chopped fresh mint
Salt and freshly ground black pepper
Lemon juice
6 sprigs of fresh mint to garnish

Grate the cucumber, peel and all. Beat the yoghurt with 150 ml (5 fl oz) of water. Stir in the cucumber, garlic (I like this soup good and garlicky, so prefer two cloves, but that's a matter of taste), lemon zest, chopped mint, salt and pepper. Taste and add a squeeze or two of lemon juice if you think it could do with sharpening up. Chill for at least 1 hour, then stir and adjust seasonings. Spoon into bowls and garnish with sprigs of mint before serving.

Cucumber Salad

This is a salad of heavenly simplicity. It's so much nicer than chucking the slices of cucumber straight into a mixed salad. I like to eat it as a first course, maybe with tinned tuna mixed with mayonnaise and capers or, for a real treat, with smoked salmon and brown bread and butter. Left-overs will keep for a day or so in the fridge and are lovely in sandwiches.

SERVES 4–6

1 large cucumber, peeled and thinly
    sliced
½ tablespoon salt
3 tablespoons white wine vinegar
    or tarragon vinegar
1 teaspoon sugar
Freshly ground black pepper
1 tablespoon chopped fresh chives

Put the sliced cucumber into a colander and sprinkle with the salt. Leave to drain for 30 minutes, then squeeze out the excess moisture with your hands. Mix with the vinegar and sugar and leave until almost ready to serve. Drain off most of the liquid, then arrange on a plate. Season with pepper and sprinkle with chives.

Three-minute Fish
with Cucumber Celery Relish

The crunchy spiced relish is a great compliment to the pure flavour of the briefly cooked fish, but there's no good reason not to serve the relish with other things. I like it with chicken, too, or even with bread and cheese.

SERVES 4–6

550–750 g (1¼–1½ lb) fillet of cod,
    halibut *or* other firm white fish
    or salmon

Olive oil for brushing
Chopped fresh chives to garnish

For the relish

½ cucumber, finely diced
Salt
2 stalks celery, finely diced
4 tablespoons rice vinegar *or* white wine
    vinegar *or* tarragon vinegar
1½ teaspoons peeled and grated fresh
    ginger

2 teaspoons caster sugar
1½ teaspoons mustard seeds
1 teaspoon dill seed
½ medium onion, very finely diced
½–1 green chilli, de-seeded and very
    finely chopped

Start with the relish. Spread the cucumber dice out in a colander and sprinkle with ½ teaspoon of salt. Leave to drain for 30 minutes, then rinse and pat dry. Mix with the celery.

Place the vinegar, ginger, sugar and seeds in a small saucepan and bring to the boil, stirring to dissolve the sugar. Simmer for 2 minutes, then add the onion and chilli, stir and draw off the heat. Mix with the cucumber and celery. Cool and leave for 30 minutes or up to 24 hours, covered and in the fridge.

Place the fish in the freezer for 10–15 minutes to firm up (not absolutely necessary, but it makes the slicing easier). Slice the fish as thinly as you can. Brush 1 large or 4 individual heatproof dishes with olive oil. Arrange the fish slices on top overlapping as little as possible. Brush with olive oil.

Pre-heat the oven to its highest setting and when everyone is gathered at table, whizz the fish into the oven for 3 minutes, or until the slices begin to turn opaque. Scatter over a few chives and serve quickly with the cool relish.

Bread and Butter Pickles

I adore these pickles, but I've often wondered how they got their name. I don't know for sure, but I suspect it is merely because they are good enough to eat neat with nothing more than thickly buttered bread. Mind you, a slice of mature cheese goes down well alongside.

Use a red onion if you can, for the colour as well as the taste. I always peel the cucumber for these pickles – they look nicer and have a better texture – but it's not absolutely necessary. The pickles can be eaten after 3 or 4 days, but they will taste even better after 3 weeks.

FILLS 2–3 450-g (1-lb) jars

1 large cucumber
1 red or white onion, very thinly sliced
1 green pepper, de-seeded and cut into strips
1½ tablespoons coarse sea salt
300 ml (10 fl oz) white wine vinegar

275 g (10 oz) caster sugar
1 tablespoon mustard seed
1 teaspoon celery seed or dill seed
5-cm (2-inch) stick of cinnamon
6 allspice berries
Pinch of cayenne pepper

Peel the cucumber if you wish and slice it into discs about 3 mm (⅛ inch) thick. Mix with the onion, pepper and salt in a bowl. Sit a plate or saucer on top, weigh down with a tin or weights and leave in the fridge for 4–12 hours or overnight. Drain, and rinse under the cold tap. Taste the cucumber and if it seems too salty rinse again. Drain thoroughly.

Place the remaining ingredients in a large saucepan and stir over a medium heat until the sugar has dissolved. Simmer for 1 minute. Add the vegetables, stir once, and bring to a bare simmer without boiling. Spoon into hot sterilized jars (see p. 61) and seal tightly. Store in a cool, dark, dry place for up to 4 months.

Brill with Melted Onions and Cucumber

The mild flavour of cucumber makes it a natural to serve with delicately flavoured fish. Here it is cooked with slowly stewed, sweet onions, to form a bed for the fillets of brill to steam on.

SERVES 4

4 large brill fillets
Salt and freshly ground black pepper
½ cucumber, cut into 1-cm (½-inch) cubes
50 g (2 oz) butter

2 large onions, thinly sliced
1 tablespoon sherry vinegar *or* red wine vinegar
½ tablespoon light muscovado sugar
1 tablespoon chopped fresh parsley

Season the brill fillets lightly with salt and pepper and set aside in the fridge. Put the cucumber into a colander and sprinkle with a teaspoon of salt. Leave for 30 minutes to drain. Rinse, then pat dry on kitchen paper.

Melt the butter in a large frying-pan. Add the onions, and stir to coat in butter. Cover (use a large plate if you don't have a lid to fit) and cook very gently for 20 minutes, stirring occasionally. Add the cucumber, vinegar, sugar and some pepper, stir again, then cook uncovered over a gentle heat for another 20 minutes until the onion is meltingly tender. Check occasionally and if absolutely necessary add a tablespoon or so of water to prevent burning.

Lay the brill fillets on top of the onion and cucumber mixture, cover the pan again, and continue cooking gently for 12–15 minutes until the fish is just cooked. Sprinkle with parsley and serve immediately.

FRUIT

Tomatoes • Aubergines • Peppers

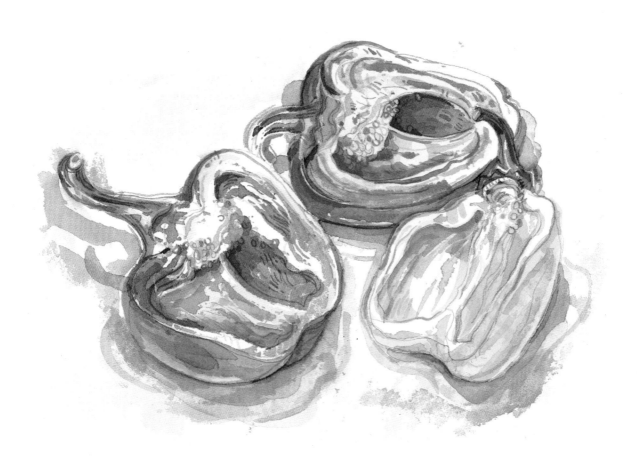

Tomatoes

Can you imagine Italian cooking without tomatoes? An impossible idea. It just wouldn't be right . . . it wouldn't be Italian. Tomatoes seem such an integral part of any Italian meal that it is hard to believe that it could ever have been otherwise. Curiously enough, tomatoes did in fact take rather a long time to catch on. They became popular in the south in the eighteenth century, particularly around Naples which is still famous for its tomatoes, but it wasn't until a hundred or so years later that the tomato finally claimed the entire boot of the country for its own.

It is only when you travel to the Mediterranean that you can really appreciate the tomato at its best. The magnificent undulating, irregular, deep red tomatoes of hot climates bear little resemblance to the poor specimens that dominate our shops and supermarkets. Visually imperfect, often all the more beautiful for that, they are bursting with intense tomatoey flavour, rich, sweet and tart, perfectly balanced in the scarlet juices that flow from them.

I've yet to be convinced that tomatoes grown in Britain can rival hot climate tomatoes. Although I believe that British tomatoes need not be as insipid and watery as most that we are offered. Gardeners know that picked full and ripe from the plant, they easily eclipse bought ones.

So why is it that bought tomatoes are more often than not so disappointing? One reason is that commercially grown tomatoes are picked under-ripe for easy transportation. They ripen off the plant, but the flavour never develops its full potential. Luckily, matters have improved lately. Some supermarkets sell tomatoes labelled 'grown for flavour' (ridiculous – what else would you grow them for? Answer: profit) which can be good. Fresh plum tomatoes are being imported from the Mediterranean, though they too are inevitably picked when immature so lose out to some degree. The only consistently excellent commercially grown tomatoes are the little cherry tomatoes, but they aren't cheap and are impractical for cooking purposes.

The moral of the story is either grow your own, or be prepared to spend a little more on 'grown for flavour' varieties. For cooking, choose tomatoes that are a deep, ripe red. What to look for in salad tomatoes is largely a question of personal taste. Slightly under-ripe tomatoes will be firmer, but more acid with a less fully developed splash of tomato-iness. This can be partly remedied with a pinch or two of sugar. Fully ripe tomatoes will have a squishier texture, but will be sweeter and more tomatoey. I usually opt for cherry tomatoes, which have the best of both texture and flavour.

Preparing Tomatoes

To skin tomatoes, simply cover them with boiling water, leave for a couple of minutes, then drain. The skin should pull away easily. If it still clings stubbornly, repeat the process. Where tomatoes are to be de-seeded, cut them in half horizontally and either scoop out the seeds with a teaspoon, or squeeze them out if the tomatoes are to be used for a sauce where they'll get crushed anyway and the odd seed isn't going to upset matters.

The length of time you cook a tomato sauce changes the flavour immeasurably. A brief spurt of high heat for a matter of 5–10 minutes or so will give a fresh, sprightly sauce, whereas slower gentle simmering for 30 minutes or more gives it a totally different character, mellow with much more depth. Either way, tomato sauce made with British tomatoes can be a stroke too acidic – you can correct this with a little sugar. To increase the fullness of flavour, add a tablespoon of tomato purée, or a glass of red wine, or even, dare I say it, a generous slurp of tomato ketchup!

Blessed with a glut of tomatoes, home-grown or on special offer in the market, the best way to preserve them is to make up a huge vat of thick sauce, with or without onion or garlic, but otherwise with little flavouring so that you can freeze it for use in any number of dishes at a later date.

Basic Tomato Sauce

This is the basic method, open to a hundred and one variations. Change the herbs, add chilli or fresh ginger, increase the garlic, omit the garlic, throw in a glass of red or white wine or the juice of an orange, leave it slightly rough and chunky, sieve or liquidize to smoothness, enrich with cream, and on and on ad infinitum.

SERVES 3–4

2 tablespoons olive oil
1 onion, chopped
1 clove garlic, peeled and chopped
450 g (1 lb) tomatoes, skinned, de-seeded and roughly chopped *or* 1 × 400 g (14 oz) tin tomatoes

1 tablespoon tomato purée
2 sprigs of fresh thyme
Chopped fresh parsley *or* torn up fresh basil leaves
Salt and freshly ground black pepper
½ teaspoon caster sugar

Warm the oil in a frying-pan and add the onion and garlic. Cook gently until tender without browning. Add tomatoes, tomato purée, thyme, parsley (if using), salt and pepper. If you are using basil it can be added at this stage, put I prefer to add it right at the end of the cooking time. Either boil hard for 5–10 minutes for a fresh-tasting sauce or simmer gently for 30 minutes until thick and rich for a mellower taste, adding a splash of water if it is drying out too quickly. Taste and adjust seasoning, adding the sugar if it is too acidic. Stir in the basil, if using.

Maria Contini's Spaghettini with Tomato Sugo

Possibly the best Italian delicatessen in the whole of Britain is to be found close to The Playhouse on the Leith side of Edinburgh. I could spend days browsing around Valvona & Crolla, with its tall, tall shelves stacked with oils and vinegars, its hams and cheeses, and the smell of lunch-time panini and pasta sauces wafting from the little kitchen upstairs, where Maria Contini cooks simple, delicious dishes to sell to a voracious stream of customers. For this classic, quick, tomato sauce you need the very best, fresh, sweet plum tomatoes. When she makes this dish Maria follows a regular ritual: while the water for the spaghettini comes to the boil, she peels and chops the tomatoes. Then, once the pasta is in the pan, she makes the sauce, knowing that it will be ready at exactly the same time as the spaghettini.

SERVES 4

350–450 g (12 oz–1 lb) spaghettini (thin spaghetti)
3 tablespoons olive oil
2 cloves garlic, peeled and sliced *or* chopped

750 g–1 kg (1½–2 lb) plum tomatoes, skinned, de-seeded and coarsely chopped
Small handful of fresh basil leaves
Salt and freshly ground black pepper
Freshly grated Parmesan cheese to serve

Bring a large pan of salted water to the boil. Add the spaghettini. As soon as the pasta is in, heat the olive oil in a large frying-pan over a brisk heat, and add the garlic. Stir for about 30 seconds, then add the tomatoes. Stir and simmer, then leave to bubble, occasionally crushing down the tomatoes, for 5 minutes or so, until they form a rough sauce. Season with salt and pepper, then roughly tear the basil leaves and scatter over the sauce. Cook for 1 minute or so more. Taste and adjust seasoning.

Drain the pasta and tip into the sauce (if there's enough room in the pan – if not, tip the sauce over the pasta in the usual way). Turn carefully, to coat, then serve with freshly grated Parmesan.

Maria Contini's Pomodori Farciti
[Stuffed Tomatoes]

Valvona & Crolla is more than just a deli — wander down to the back of the shop where the shelves groan with hundreds of bottles of wine, and you find a stand piled high with the best quality fresh vegetables and wild mushrooms in season. In summer there will be two types of tomatoes — glossy red plum tomatoes for sauces and salads and craggy beef tomatoes for stuffing. Neither will necessarily be perfect looking, but you can bet that the flavour will be outstanding.

Maria Contini uses medium-sized beef tomatoes for this recipe. She likes to use French bread, crust and all, for the breadcrumbs, but all the other ingredients come straight from the shop. If you use salted capers, as Maria does, rinse first and add salt to the stuffing with caution. Serve as a side dish, or a first course.

SERVES 4

4 beef tomatoes
100 g (4 oz) slightly stale breadcrumbs
  (use crust as well)
2 large cloves garlic, peeled and finely
  chopped
Generous handful of fresh parsley, finely
  chopped

1 tablespoon capers, roughly chopped
Salt and freshly ground black pepper
5 tablespoons extra virgin olive oil
50 g (2 oz) freshly grated Parmesan
  cheese

Remove the stalks of the tomatoes, and cut each tomato in half horizontally. Scoop out the insides and reserve. Leave the tomato shells upside-down to drain for 15 minutes or so.

Pre-heat the oven to gas mark 5, 375°F (190°C). Mix the breadcrumbs with the garlic, parsley, capers and about 3 tablespoons of the juicy bit of the insides of the tomatoes, breaking

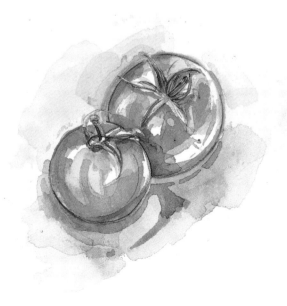

up any large lumps of flesh. Season with salt and pepper and mix in just enough of the olive oil to moisten – about 3 tablespoons. Stuff the tomatoes with this mixture and sit in an oiled baking dish. Sprinkle over the Parmesan, then drizzle over a final 2 tablespoons of olive oil. Bake for about 20 minutes, until lightly browned and sizzling. Serve hot or warm.

Pappa al Pomodoro
[Bread and Tomato Soup]

This marvellous, robust bread and tomato soup from Tuscany is only worth making if you use good-quality country-style bread. It is thick and filling so serve in small quantities. I like it best hot, but it can be served cold too, though you may have to add extra stock to thin it down.

SERVES 6–8

350 g (12 oz) stale bread with crusts, thickly sliced
1 large onion, chopped
150 ml (5 fl oz) olive oil
4 cloves garlic, peeled and finely chopped

1 kg (2 lb) ripe tomatoes, skinned and roughly chopped
Salt and freshly ground black pepper
1.5 litres (2½ pints) light chicken *or* vegetable stock
1 small bunch of fresh basil, shredded

To serve
Extra virgin olive oil
Freshly grated Parmesan (*optional*)

Pre-heat the oven to gas mark 2, 300°F (150°C).

Spread the bread out on a baking sheet and dry in the oven for 10–15 minutes. Break into pieces.

Fry the onion in 2 tablespoons of olive oil until just tender. Add the garlic and raise the heat slightly. As soon as the garlic begins to brown add the tomatoes, salt and pepper. Simmer for 10 minutes. Cool slightly, then pass through the fine plate of a mouli-légumes or liquidize and sieve.

Bring the stock up to the boil and add the puréed tomato mixture, bread, remaining olive oil, basil, salt and pepper. Simmer for 20–30 minutes, stirring occasionally, until the soup is very thick. Taste and adjust seasonings. Serve hot or cold, with a drizzle of olive oil and, if you wish, a scattering of Parmesan.

Moroccan Salad

Cumin is the spice that I associate most strongly with Morocco. It goes into all manner of dishes, hot and cold, lending its warm aromatic scent. It is added to salads as well as cooked dishes, and it is what makes this salad of diced tomato and grilled green pepper so special.

SERVES 4–6

2 large green peppers
450 g (1 lb) ripe tomatoes, skinned,
    de-seeded and chopped

For the dressing

1 tablespoon lemon juice
3 tablespoons extra virgin olive oil
1 large clove garlic, peeled and crushed
½ teaspoon ground cumin

2 tablespoons finely chopped fresh
    parsley *or* a mixture of parsley and
    fresh coriander
Salt and freshly ground black pepper

Quarter the peppers and remove the seeds. Grill, skin-side to heat, until blackened and blistered. Drop into a plastic bag, knot the ends and leave until cool enough to handle. Strip off the skin, then cut the peppers into small pieces. Mix with the tomatoes and any juice given out by the peppers.

    To make the dressing mix all the ingredients. Toss with the tomatoes and peppers. Serve at room temperature.

Michel Guérard's Tarte Fine
à la Tomate et au Pistou

A 'tarte fine' is a thin disc of puff pastry, covered with a savoury or sweet filling and baked quickly in a hot oven. This recipe, from French chef, Michel Guérard, pairs the thin crisp pastry with tomatoes, basil and olive oil. With richly flavoured tomatoes, it is the most heavenly first course. The only drawback is that you will probably have to cook the 'tartes fines' in relays, unless you have an extremely large oven.

SERVES 6

2 tablespoons finely chopped fresh basil
120 ml (4 fl oz) extra virgin olive oil
2 tablespoons tomato purée
450 g (1 lb) puff pastry
6 ripe, medium-sized tomatoes

Salt and freshly ground black pepper
Sugar
½ teaspoon fresh thyme leaves
12 extra basil leaves, roughly torn up

Mix the chopped basil with 1½ tablespoons of the olive oil and set aside for 5–10 minutes, then mix with the tomato purée. Roll out the puff pastry very thinly (it's probably easiest to do this in 2 halves) and cut out six 20-cm (8-inch) diameter circles. Prick all over with a fork

---

OVERLEAF *Michel Guérard's Tarte Fine à la Tomate et au Pistou*

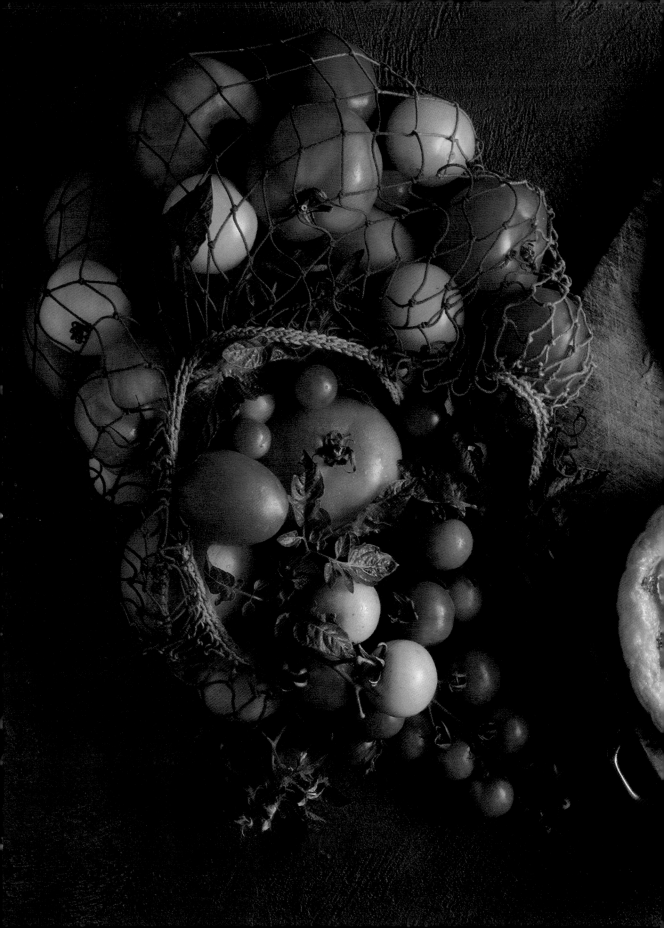

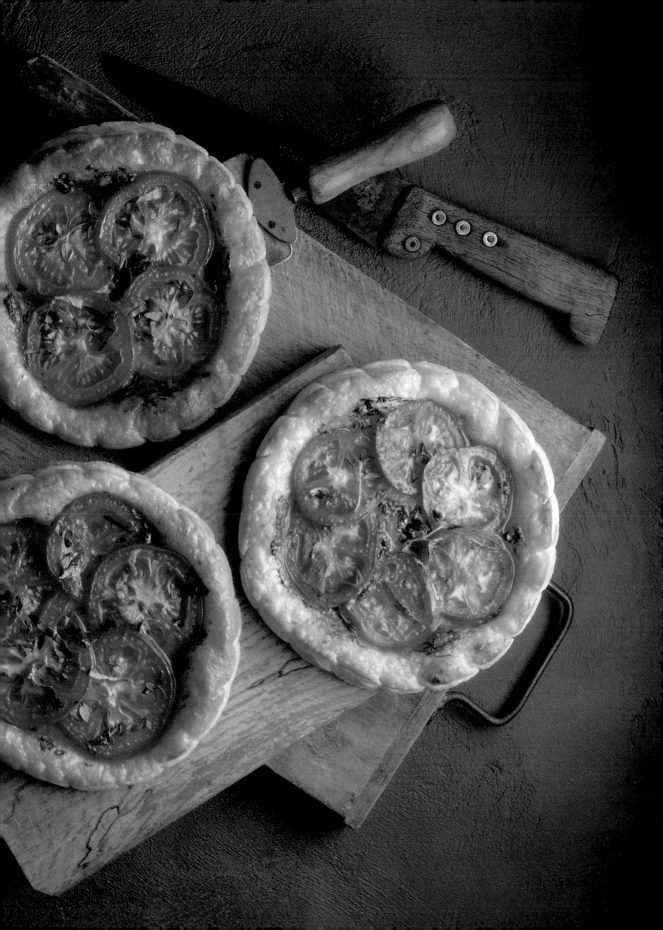

and lay them on oiled baking sheets. Spread the basil and tomato purée mixture over the circles, using a brush, leaving a 1-cm (½-inch) border all the way round the edges.

Pre-heat the oven to gas mark 8, 450°F (230°C). Slice the tomatoes as thinly as you can. Discard the seeds and juice. Arrange the tomato rings on the pastry. Season with salt, pepper and a little sugar. Scatter over the thyme. Bake in the oven. After 5 minutes, brush the tarts generously with olive oil and return to the oven for a final 5–8 minutes until nicely browned. Serve immediately, scattered with a few torn up basil leaves.

Tomato and Pepper Summer Pudding

Made in much the same way as a sweet summer pudding, this savoury version filled with tomatoes and peppers is a perfect dish for a lazy summer lunch. The 'pudding' has to be made at least 12 hours, preferably 24 hours, in advance. It looks pretty too, a glowing red mound decorated with fresh green herbs.

SERVES 4 as a main course, 6–8 as a first course

6–10 thin slices slightly stale white
    bread, crusts removed

Fresh herbs (parsley and basil) to
    decorate

For the filling

2 onions, chopped
2 cloves garlic, peeled and chopped
1 red pepper, de-seeded and cut into
    strips
1 green pepper, de-seeded and cut into
    strips
3 tablespoons olive oil
2 × 400 g (14 oz) tins tomatoes
    or 1 kg (2 lb) fresh tomatoes,
    skinned and roughly chopped

2 tablespoons tomato purée
3 sprigs of fresh thyme *or* 1 teaspoon
    dried
1 tablespoon red wine vinegar
2 teaspoons sugar
Salt and freshly ground black pepper

Make the filling first. Cook the onions, garlic and peppers gently in the oil until tender. Add all the remaining ingredients and simmer until fairly thick. Taste and adjust seasoning. Remove the thyme sprigs.

Line a 900-ml–1.2 litre (1½–2 pint) pudding basin with the bread, trimming so that it fits in snugly with no gaps but no overlaps either. Fill with the tomato and pepper mixture and cover with bread trimmed to fit. Lay a plate or large saucer on top and weigh down with tins or metal weights. Leave overnight in the fridge.

Just before serving remove weight and plate, and cover the pudding with a shallow serving dish. Invert, give it a firm shake and the pudding should slip nicely out onto the plate.

Aubergines

That aubergines and tomatoes should belong to the same botanical family seems reasonable enough. But that they should be first cousins to potatoes and deadly nightshade seems far more unlikely. Surely these two must be cuckoos in the Solanaceae family nest? It's only on the rare occasion when you see the fruit of a potato plant that the kinship becomes obvious. It looks just like a small, green immature tomato or aubergine, round and glossy with a tough green calyx where it meets the stalk. And, like deadly nightshade, it is highly poisonous. The family connections are all there.

Cousins they may be, but unlike the New World potato and tomato, the origins of the aubergine lie right across on the other side of the globe, in Asia. They reached Europe, probably via Africa, over a hundred years before Columbus returned with his vegetable haul. Now they seem one of the most essential and fundamental of Mediterranean vegetables.

Their successful and rapid colonization of the countries that fringe the Mediterranean sea is remarkable only for its speed. Aubergines grow easily and abundantly in hot climates, but more important than that is, I suspect, their unique culinary qualities. The thing about aubergines is that they slot comfortably into any style of cooking. Though the flavour is clearly defined, it is restrained enough to take on other more powerful flavours without losing identity. In fact it begs for big flavours – spices, herbs, chillies, olive oil, garlic. It blends, it absorbs, it harmonizes. The texture is important too. Like a sponge, aubergine sucks in oil and flavourings, cooking down to a wonderfully melting creaminess, as good cold as hot. There's nothing else quite like it.

Though the south of Italy boastfully claims more aubergine recipes than any other region of the world, their range is nonetheless limited. Travel back towards aubergines' homeland, and all along the route you come across marvellous ways of using them to their utmost. In the Middle East they are warmly, aromatically spiced, and when you reach Asia, in particular India (where they are called Brinjal) and China, they are transformed into the most exotic of dishes.

Preparing Aubergines

Though you can cook aubergines just as they are, you would be well advised to salt them first. Salt draws out (or 'degorges') some of their juices and improves the flavour no end. Unsalted aubergines may have what is usually described as a bitter flavour, though that's not really quite the right word. It's more tinny than bitter, an aftertaste rather than an upfront impression. Salted aubergines will also absorb less oil, a bonus, both calorie- and pocket-wise, when they are to be fried, and they develop a more voluptuous texture.

In most instances, salting is a simple matter – just sprinkle the cut aubergines with salt and leave them alone for at least 30 minutes, preferably a full hour, then either wipe clean, or rinse and pat dry. When small aubergines are to be used whole, they should be pierced first with a skewer and left to soak for an hour or two in salted water. Obviously, when a recipe calls for a large aubergine to be grilled or baked whole, neither approach is going to work. Here the answer is to drain the flesh of the cooked aubergine thoroughly, squeezing out as much of the liquid as possible.

Once cut, aubergine will start to turn brown. Unsightly, perhaps, but there's little point in taking steps to prevent it, as the flesh darkens anyway as it cooks.

By and large, aubergines are not eaten raw, though the Stylianous, who grow aubergines in North London and gave me the recipe opposite, do add raw aubergine to their Greek salad. I tried a piece, and have to admit that it was not much to my taste. Besides, it's not advisable to eat raw aubergine in any quantity as it contains a small amount of toxic solanine, which is only eliminated by heat.

Aubergines like oil, and no doubt about it. Even salted aubergines drink up a fair quantity in the frying-pan. This is partly what makes the smoothness of fried aubergines so delicious, but over-indulge and you're bound to feel queasy. Still, you don't have to fry them. Grilled slices of aubergine are deliciously smoky, and all they need is a quick brushing with oil before they hit the heat. Where the aubergine slices are to be incorporated into a substantial dish, such as moussaka, they can be steamed (but not boiled, as they tend to become watery and mushy), though the no-oil-at-all approach makes aubergine too worthy for simpler dishes.

Maria Stylianou's Aubergine Casserole

Maria Stylianou left Greece when she was a young woman to work as a nanny in Britain. She met her Cypriot husband, Anastasis, here, and now they live in North London. But every sunny day, they return to their own corner of Cyprus – an allotment in Muswell Hill.

There are quince and plum trees, a Cypriot apple tree, patches of coriander and vegetables and a greenhouse packed full of aubergine, pepper and melon plants. The Stylianous sit under a canopy of vine leaves, surrounded by a hedge of scented roses, to eat the meals that Maria prepares on the two-ring camping gas stove in the make-shift 'living-room' shed.

This casserole of aubergine, potato and tomato is one that reminds them of home. It's a summer dish, filling and delicious, and cheap too when you grow your own vegetables. I like it hot, but the Stylianous told me firmly that it should be eaten cold, with plenty of crusty Greek bread to mop up the juices.

SERVES 4

3 medium aubergines
Salt
4 medium to large potatoes
120 ml (4 fl oz) olive oil
2 cloves garlic, peeled and roughly
  chopped

2–3 bay leaves
2 onions, chopped
2 large beef tomatoes, skinned and
  chopped
½ tablespoon sugar
Salt and freshly ground black pepper

Cut the aubergines into quarters lengthwise, then cut each quarter in half. Spread out in a colander and sprinkle with salt. Leave for 30 minutes or so to drain. Wipe dry.

Peel the potatoes and cut into large chunks. In a large frying-pan fry the potatoes in the olive oil over a moderate heat until golden brown and three-quarters cooked. Transfer them to a flameproof casserole or large saucepan.

Fry the aubergine in the same oil until tender and browned. Lay the aubergines on top of the potatoes. Add 1 clove of garlic and the bay leaves.

Fry the onions and remaining garlic gently in 2 tablespoons of the oil until tender and lightly browned. Add the tomatoes and sugar, salt and pepper. Simmer gently for 15 minutes. Pour over the aubergines and potatoes. Cover, leaving a small gap for steam to escape, and simmer gently for 20–30 minutes stirring occasionally until the potatoes are cooked and sauce is thick. Serve hot or cold.

Poor Man's Caviar

Lucky poor man, even if he can't afford the real thing. If you chop the aubergine finely, this does have a vague visual resemblance to pearly grey caviar, though I prefer the texture when it's whizzed smooth in the blender. Either way, the taste is delicious but not at all like caviar.

Grilled aubergine, particularly if it is grilled over charcoal, has a wonderful smoky flavour, though if it is more convenient, oven-baked aubergine still works well.

SERVES 3–4 as a first course

1 large aubergine
2 tablespoons olive oil
2 tablespoons chopped fresh parsley
1–2 cloves garlic, peeled and crushed
½ teaspoon ground cumin

Pinch of chilli powder
Juice of ½–1 lemon
Salt and freshly ground black pepper
Pitta bread or toast to serve

Either grill the aubergine whole, turning frequently until the skin is blackened and blistered and the aubergine is very soft, or bake the aubergine in a very hot oven until very soft – about 20–30 minutes. Cool for a few minutes until you can bear to handle it. Cut in half lengthways and either pull the charred skin off or scrape the flesh out. Place flesh in a colander and squeeze with your hands to expel the bitter juices.

Chop roughly and then whizz in a blender, gradually adding all the remaining ingredients. When you get to the lemon juice, add only enough to balance out the flavours and take the edge off the richness of the purée. Serve with warm pitta bread or toast.

Grilled Aubergine Salad

A favourite salad of mine – a dark gleaming mass of aubergines, smoky and rich with a garlicky hiss. Grilled aubergine slices, simply salted, then brushed with oil and seasoned before grilling, are good hot too.

SERVES 6

2 large aubergines
Salt
2–3 tablespoons chopped mixed herbs –
    fresh parsley, fresh basil
    and/or fresh chives

For the dressing

1½ tablespoons white or red wine
    vinegar
1–2 cloves garlic, peeled and crushed
Salt and freshly ground black pepper
7 tablespoons extra virgin olive oil

To make the dressing, mix the vinegar with the garlic, pepper and a little salt. Whisk in the olive oil a tablespoon at a time.

Slice the aubergines into 1-cm (½-inch) thick discs. Sprinkle lightly with salt and leave for 30 minutes to 1 hour. Wipe dry. Toss with half the dressing. Grill, close to the heat, until browned on both sides. Toss with enough of the remaining dressing to moisten, then leave to cool. Toss with the chopped herbs and serve.

Fish-fragrant Aubergine

No fish at all in this Chinese recipe, despite the name. The aubergine is cooked with the flavourings that are often used with fish – hence fish-fragrant. Fish or no fish, it's a marvellous way to cook aubergine, spiced and melting and quite irresistible. Be warned though, when the chilli hits the hot oil, the fumes are forceful enough to make you cough and splutter.

Sichuan pepper is not a true pepper at all, but it does have a tingly, numbing heat and a marvellous incense-like aroma. Some larger supermarkets and good delicatessens, and all oriental food shops will stock it. It's well worth hunting out, though black pepper can stand in at a pinch in this recipe.

SERVES 3–4

1 very large aubergine or 2 small ones
1 teaspoon salt
2 dried red chillies
Sunflower or vegetable oil for deep-frying
3 spring onions, sliced
2 cloves garlic, peeled and finely chopped
1-cm (½-inch) piece of fresh ginger, peeled and finely chopped

1 tablespoon soy sauce
1 teaspoon sugar
Large pinch of freshly ground Sichuan *or* black pepper
1 tablespoon rice vinegar *or* white wine vinegar
1 teaspoon sesame oil

Cut the aubergine into slices about 2.5 cm (1 inch) thick. Cut each slice into diamond-shaped chunks. Spread out in a colander and sprinkle with a teaspoon of salt. Leave to drain for 30 minutes. Rinse under the cold tap, drain and pat dry on kitchen paper. Soak the chillies in warm water for 15 minutes, then cut each one into 3 pieces, discarding the seeds.

Heat enough oil in a wok to deep-fry the aubergine chunks. When it's just smoking add the aubergine and deep-fry for 3–4 minutes until golden brown. Scoop out and drain on kitchen paper. Pour off all but 1 tablespoon of the oil. Re-heat and add the chilli, spring onions, garlic and ginger. Stir-fry for 30 seconds. Add the aubergine and toss. Now add all the remaining ingredients except the sesame oil. Stir-fry for a further 1–2 minutes. Stir in the sesame oil and serve.

Pasta Alla *Norma*

Vincenzo Bellini, composer of the opera Norma, *was a native of Catania in Sicily. In his home town this dish of pasta with aubergine and tomato has been rechristened in his honour, though it is known by other names throughout the island.*

Serves 4

1 large aubergine
Salt
2–3 cloves garlic, peeled and chopped
Olive oil for frying
750 g (1½ lb) ripe tomatoes, skinned,
    de-seeded, and chopped
Salt and freshly ground black pepper

400–450 g (14–16 oz) spaghetti
3 tablespoons grated ricotta salata
    or Pecorino or Parmesan cheese
Handful of fresh basil leaves, roughly
    torn up
Extra ricotta salata or Pecorino or
    Parmesan cheese to serve

Slice the aubergine into 1-cm (½-inch) discs and cut into 1-cm (½-inch) wide strips. Spread out in a colander and sprinkle with salt. Leave to drain for an hour, then rinse and pat dry.

Fry the garlic gently in 4 tablespoons olive oil until beginning to colour. Add the tomatoes, salt and pepper and simmer for 15 minutes or so to make a thick tomato sauce. Reheat when needed.

Bring a large pan of salted water to the boil and add the spaghetti. Boil until *al dente*. While the spaghetti is cooking, heat a generous layer of olive oil in a wide frying-pan, and fry the aubergine until browned, in 2 batches if necessary. Drain on kitchen paper.

Drain the spaghetti and tip into a large serving bowl. Add the hot tomato sauce, the ricotta salata or Pecorino or Parmesan, and the basil. Toss quickly. Top with the fried aubergine and serve with extra cheese to hand round.

Baked Aubergine with Tomato and Mozzarella

This is a rustically elegant first course, again from Italy as so many good aubergine recipes are. It can all be prepared in advance, ready to go into the oven as soon as your guests arrive.

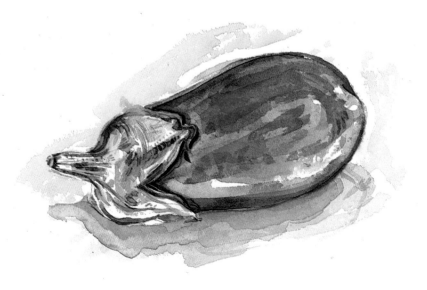

SERVES 4 as a first course

1 large aubergine
Salt
½ ball of Mozzarella cheese (about
    65 g/2½ oz), diced

Olive oil
Salt and freshly ground black pepper
8 fresh basil leaves

For the sauce

1 onion, finely chopped
2 cloves garlic, peeled and finely
    chopped
1 tablespoon finely chopped fresh
    parsley
2 sprigs fresh thyme *or* ½ teaspoon dried

2 tablespoons olive oil
1 × 400 g (14 oz) tin chopped
    tomatoes
1 tablespoon tomato purée
½ teaspoon sugar
Salt and freshly ground black pepper

Cut the aubergine into 8 thick discs, discarding the ends. Spread out on a plate and sprinkle lightly with salt. Leave for at least 30 minutes, preferably a full hour, to exude the bitter juices. Then wipe clean.

While the aubergine is being salted, make the tomato sauce. Cook the onion, garlic, parsley and thyme gently in the oil until tender, without browning. Add the remaining sauce ingredients, bring to the boil, and cook hard until good and thick with no trace of wateriness. Taste and adjust seasoning.

Pre-heat the oven to gas mark 4, 350°F (180°C). Oil an ovenproof baking dish generously. Lay the aubergine slices in it in a single layer without overlapping. Brush with more olive oil and cover with foil. Bake for 30 minutes. Take out of the oven, uncover, and spread each slice thickly with tomato sauce – you won't use it all up, so save the rest to serve warm or cold with lunch or supper on another day.

Dot a few cubes of Mozzarella on each slice, drizzle a generous tablespoon of olive oil over the slices, season with salt and pepper and return to the oven, uncovered, for a further 15 minutes. Serve 2 slices per person, jauntily topped with a basil leaf a piece.

Melanzane Sott'olio
[Aubergines Preserved in Olive Oil]

This is a preserve I'm particularly fond of – strips of aubergine preserved in oil with a handful of aromatics. As they sit in their jars, the purple of the skins gradually creeps into the pale flesh. A beautiful sight. Serve them as part of an antipasto with plates of salami, cured ham, olives, cheese, and plenty of crusty bread.

OVERLEAF *Baked Aubergine with Tomato and Mozzarella*

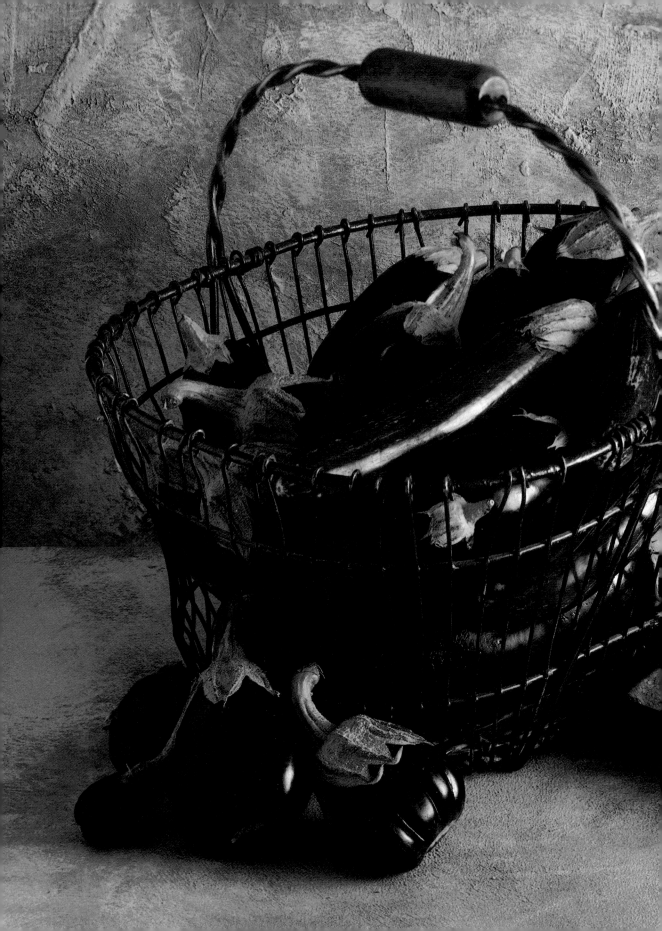

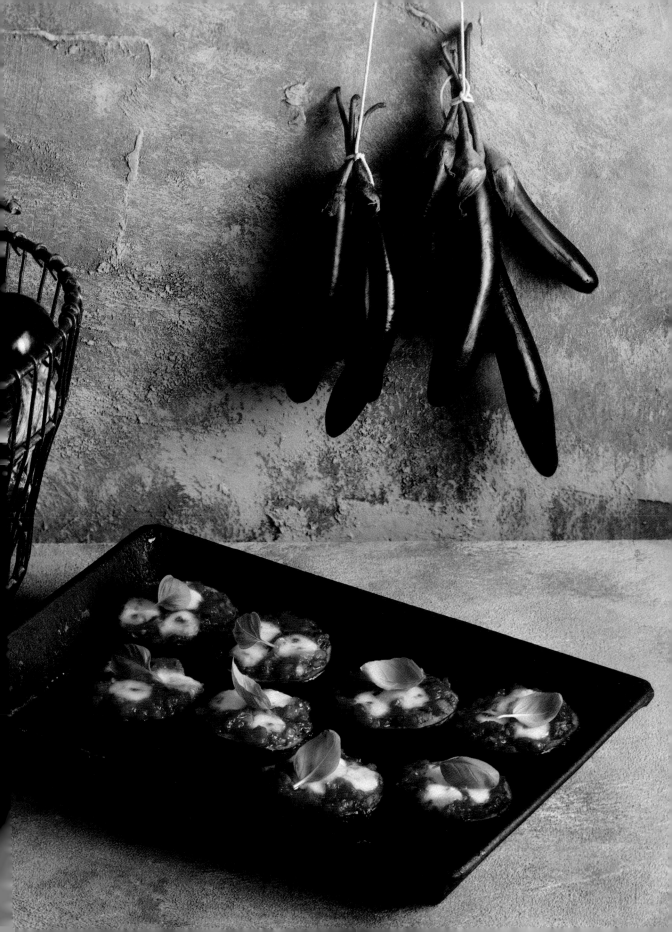

Serves 6–8

450 g (1 lb) aubergine
Salt
150 ml (5 fl oz) white wine vinegar
150–200 ml (5–7 fl oz) extra virgin
   olive oil
150–200 ml (5–7 fl oz) sunflower oil

4 cloves garlic, peeled and finely
   chopped
1–3 fresh red chillies, finely chopped
Leaves of 2 sprigs of fresh thyme
   or ½ teaspoon dried

Slice the aubergine into discs about 2.5 cm (1 inch) thick, and then into strips 2.5 cm (1 inch) wide. Layer in a large colander, sprinkling each layer with salt. Set aside for 4 hours, turning occasionally. Rinse under the cold tap.

Place the aubergine strips in a pan with the vinegar and just enough water to cover. Bring to the boil and simmer gently for 5–10 minutes until tender. Drain thoroughly and pat dry with kitchen paper.

Mix 150 ml (5 fl oz) olive oil with an equal quantity of sunflower oil. Mix garlic, chilli and thyme together. Into a sterilized preserving jar (see page 61) pour enough of the oil mixture to cover the base. Sprinkle with a little of the garlic, chilli and thyme mixture. Add a layer of aubergines, sprinkle with a little more of the garlic, chilli and thyme, and pour in enough oil to cover. Repeat until all aubergine is used up, covering the final layer generously with oil. You may find that you need a little extra oil.

Cover loosely and leave to stand in a cool place for 1–2 hours to settle. If necessary add more oil to cover completely. Seal tightly and keep in a cool, dry, dark place for at least a week and up to 6 months.

Claudia Roden's
Sweet Aubergine Preserve

The novelist Paul Bailey first introduced me to this unlikely but marvellous sweet aubergine preserve from Claudia Roden's New Book of Middle Eastern Food *(Penguin). It is usually made with tiny whole aubergines, but I prefer this version made with cubed aubergine. It is lovely on toast, but even better served as a pudding with plenty of yoghurt.*

Makes about 1.75 kg (4 lb)

1 kg (2 lb) aubergines
Salt
1 kg (2 lb) sugar
1–2 teaspoons whole cloves
½ teaspoon ground ginger
Juice of ½ lemon

Cut the aubergines into 2-cm (¾-inch) cubes. Spread out in a colander and sprinkle with salt. Leave for an hour, then press to squeeze out juice, and rinse in cold water. Poach in unsalted water for 5–10 minutes until tender. Drain thoroughly.

Put the sugar into a large saucepan with 900 ml (1½ pints) water, the spices and lemon juice. Bring slowly to the boil, stirring to dissolve the sugar. Add the aubergine and simmer for about 1 hour until the aubergines are thoroughly impregnated with sugar and meltingly tender. Cool. Spoon the aubergines into sterilized jars (see page 61) and cover with the syrup which should be thick enough to coat a spoon. If not, reduce it by boiling fast, then pour over the aubergines. Seal and label. Store in a cool, dark, dry place for up to 6 months.

Escalivada

My first taste of escalivada was in a beach-side restaurant in Barcelona. It was a balmy, warm spring day and the meal was of blissful perfect simplicity – this salad of grilled vegetables, followed by a plate of grilled seafood and glasses of chilled white wine. Who could ask for more?

So, when the next sunny day comes along, set up the barbecue, or heat the grill, and make a big dish full of escalivada. Grilling the individual vegetables takes a little time as you may have to do it in batches, but you will be amply rewarded.

SERVES 6

4 small onions	Extra virgin olive oil
1 aubergine	Salt and freshly ground black pepper
4 red peppers	Fresh parsley, chopped
2 cloves garlic, peeled and finely chopped	2 hard-boiled eggs, shelled and quartered

Heat your grill thoroughly. Pull any loose, papery skin off the onions and trim back stalks and roots. Arrange whole onions, aubergine and peppers on the grill rack, and grill about 5 cm (2 inches) from the heat, turning when outer skins are charred and crisp. Remove from the rack when they are charred all over and softened. Drop each type of vegetable into a separate plastic bag, knot and leave for 5–10 minutes, until just cool enough to handle.

Pull the skin off the aubergine and cut the flesh into long strips. Drain off the bitter juices in a colander whilst you prepare the other vegetables. Skin the peppers and cut into long strips. Peel the onions, and cut into eighths. Arrange on a serving plate, in separate bands, touching but not mixing or overlapping. Scatter the garlic over them, and drizzle a generous amount of olive oil over the vegetables. Season lightly and leave to cool.

Just before serving, scatter with a little chopped parsley, and arrange quarters of hard-boiled eggs on the bed of vegetables.

Peppers

Why do we call sweet peppers by that name when they bear no resemblance or botanical kinship to peppercorns proper? It can be downright confusing. Wouldn't it be easier if we could retrain ourselves to think of them as capsicums? Food writers occasionally try it out for size, but the more usual 'peppers' clings tenaciously. We have Columbus and the conquistadores to blame for the linguistic muddle. In the fifteenth and sixteenth centuries spices, and pepper in particular, were precious commodities. Instead of a new route to the rich spices of the Orient, the Spanish explorers discovered a strange, fertile land – the Americas. They found tomatoes, potatoes and corn, all fascinating curiosities, but of no obvious value (at the time . . .). The determined search for pepper led them to another plant, the chilli. In its primitive form, the tiny round fruit might well have looked somewhat akin to fresh peppercorns on the vine. They certainly tasted hot. They were carried back in triumph to the Old World and hopefully christened 'pimiento', after the Spanish name for black pepper. Hence peppers in English, though curiously the name is now more commonly used for sweet peppers than the original hot chillies. (The word chilli comes from the Nahuatl Indian language.)

It took a long time for sweet peppers to come in any quantity to our shores. They are a post-war phenomenon, popularized by the late Elizabeth David and the food writers that followed her. Now they are commonplace, sold in every greengrocery and supermarket, grown on windowsills and in greenhouses. Their appeal is obvious – they might have been designed to hang from the branches of Christmas trees with their brightly coloured polished skins.

There's a veritable rainbow of peppers to be had these days. Besides red and green, there's yellow, orange and dark, black-purple-skinned types. Occasionally the pale-green, conical banana or Hungarian wax pepper puts in an appearance too. In flavour they boil down to a choice of two. Green ones have a more savoury taste – not so surprising as they are merely unripened red (or yellow or orange) peppers. Fully ripened red, orange and yellow peppers are sweeter. The remarkable purple peppers are a bit of a disappointment; the moment you cook them the brooding colour fades to a murky green. Save them for a bit of dark drama in a salad.

Preparing Peppers

Never buy peppers that are wrinkled with damp, squishy patches. They are well past their sell-by date and shopkeepers who sell them should be ashamed. Basic preparation is straightforward and obvious. Just remove the stalk and seeds, and cut them into whatever shapes you need.

Though I like the fresh, juicy taste of raw peppers in salads and salsas, I really prefer them cooked. Heat induces a vast improvement in the flavour, making it more complex and interesting. Top in my league of pepper cooking methods is grilling and skinning which gives them the most voluptuous of textures. This is a technique used in several of the recipes that follow. Should you ever come across the words '1 pepper, skinned' in a list of ingredients, it doesn't mean that you should get out the vegetable peeler and discard half the pepper, but that they should be grilled to loosen the skin.

Frying peppers, often followed by braising, produces another new taste and texture. The Italians have peperonata, fried peppers finished with tomatoes. It's much the same as the Spanish pisto on p. 174, minus the eggs, and using parsley or basil instead of dried mixed herbs. Peppers are obvious candidates for stuffing – their alternative name capsicum, from their Latin botanical name, is believed to come from the Latin, *capsa*, a box. They can be baked from raw, complete with filling, but I find that straight baked peppers can have a slightly tinny taste, so I usually blanch them briefly first, which keeps them sweet and pure and shortens the cooking time.

Margaret's Fried Eggs
with Grilled Peppers

This idea for a light lunch or supper was given to me by Margaret Hobbs who set up the delicatessen beside the Pont de la Tour restaurant in London. She made it with the pancetta bread they sell there, but any good quality bread can be used instead. The combination of crisp bread, soft egg, and sweet grilled peppers is a triumph.

SERVES 2

1 large red pepper
2 thick slices good bread
Olive oil for frying
2 eggs

Dash of balsamic vinegar *or* sherry vinegar
4 large fresh basil leaves, torn up, to garnish
Salt and freshly ground black pepper

Quarter the pepper and remove stalk, seeds and white membrane. Grill, skin-side close to heat, until skin is blackened and blistered. Drop into a plastic bag, knot and leave until cool enough to handle. Strip off skin, and then cut into strips. Reserve along with any juice.

Stamp or cut a 6-cm (2½-inch) circle out of the centre of each slice of bread. Heat about 2 tablespoons of olive oil in a saucepan large enough to take the 2 slices of bread. Fry the bread on both sides until golden brown. Carefully break an egg into the central hole in each slice, holding the slice down for a few seconds to prevent any egg seeping out underneath. Reduce the heat, and cover pan. Leave to cook for 7–10 minutes, until the egg white is just set.

A few minutes before the eggs are done, warm the pepper strips and their juices with about ½ tablespoon of olive oil in a small saucepan. As soon as the eggs are ready, arrange the bread and egg slices on 2 plates. Stir a dash of balsamic vinegar, salt and pepper into the peppers, and pile the mixture on top of the slices. Scatter with basil leaves and serve.

Grilled Pepper Salad

Grilled peppers have the most wonderful, voluptuous texture and a heavenly smoky sweetness. They make one of the best of all salads, served perhaps as an antipasto, alongside a plate of salamis and cured hams and with plenty of good bread to mop up the juices. This is how you prepare them.

Quarter as many peppers – green, red and yellow – as you need (one will serve 2–3 people) and remove the seeds. Pre-heat the grill (or barbecue) thoroughly. Grill the peppers skin-side close to the heat, until the skins are thoroughly blackened and blistered. Drop into a plastic bag, knot the ends and leave until the peppers are cool enough to handle. The captured steam loosens the skins, so that they will strip off easily.

Once skinned, cut the peppers into strips and place in a dish with any juice they have given out. Drizzle over some olive oil, add a little crushed garlic if you wish, then season with salt and freshly ground black pepper. Leave to cool and scatter over a little chopped fresh parsley, or roughly torn up basil leaves.

Anchovy fillets, halved lengthways, or pitted black olives, roughly sliced, or strips of sun-dried tomato preserved in olive oil are all good additions, their saltiness highlighting the sweetness of the grilled peppers. A teaspoon or so of Balsamic vinegar adds a mellow hint of sharpness.

Sautéed Peppers with Balsamic Vinegar

A quick, easy way to cook peppers, bringing out their sweetness to the full. The sautéed peppers can be served hot or cold, as a side dish, hors d'œuvre or even on hot pasta.

SERVES 4

3 tablespoons olive oil
1 large red onion, sliced
1 red pepper, de-seeded and cut into
1-cm (½-inch) wide strips
1 green pepper, de-seeded and cut into
1-cm (½-inch) wide strips

1 clove garlic, peeled and finely
chopped
½ teaspoon ground coriander
½ tablespoon balsamic vinegar
Salt and freshly ground black pepper

Heat the oil over a moderate heat in a wide frying-pan. Add the onion and fry over a gentle heat, stirring occasionally, for 10 minutes. Raise the heat and add the peppers and sauté briskly until tender and patched with brown. Add the garlic and coriander and continue to fry for a further 2 minutes. Tip into a dish and season with balsamic vinegar, salt and pepper. Serve.

Chickpeas with Chorizo and Peppers

This is a more substantial way of using sautéed peppers, stewed with chickpeas and spicy Spanish chorizo sausage (from good delicatessens). If you are really short of time, or forget to put the dried chickpeas to soak, you can substitute 450 g (1 lb) drained weight of tinned chickpeas, though they have an inferior texture and taste.

SERVES 4

225 g (8 oz) dried chickpeas, soaked
overnight
Generous pinch of saffron threads
2 cloves garlic, peeled and chopped
1 onion, chopped
1 red pepper, de-seeded and cut into
strips
1 green pepper, de-seeded and cut into
strips

2 tablespoons olive oil
225 g (8 oz) chorizo, skinned and
thickly sliced
1 rounded tablespoon chopped fresh
parsley
150 ml (5 fl oz) vegetable *or* light
chicken stock
Salt and freshly ground black pepper

Drain the chickpeas and rinse. Boil in unsalted water until tender. Drain well. Mix the saffron threads with a tablespoon of warm water and leave to steep.

Fry the garlic, onion, red and green pepper in the oil until tender, without browning. Raise the heat slightly and add the chorizo. Fry until it begins to brown. Now add the chickpeas, and all the remaining ingredients including the saffron and its water. Simmer for 10 minutes, stirring occasionally, until most of the liquid has evaporated. Taste and adjust seasoning, then serve.

OVERLEAF *Chickpeas with Chorizo and Peppers*

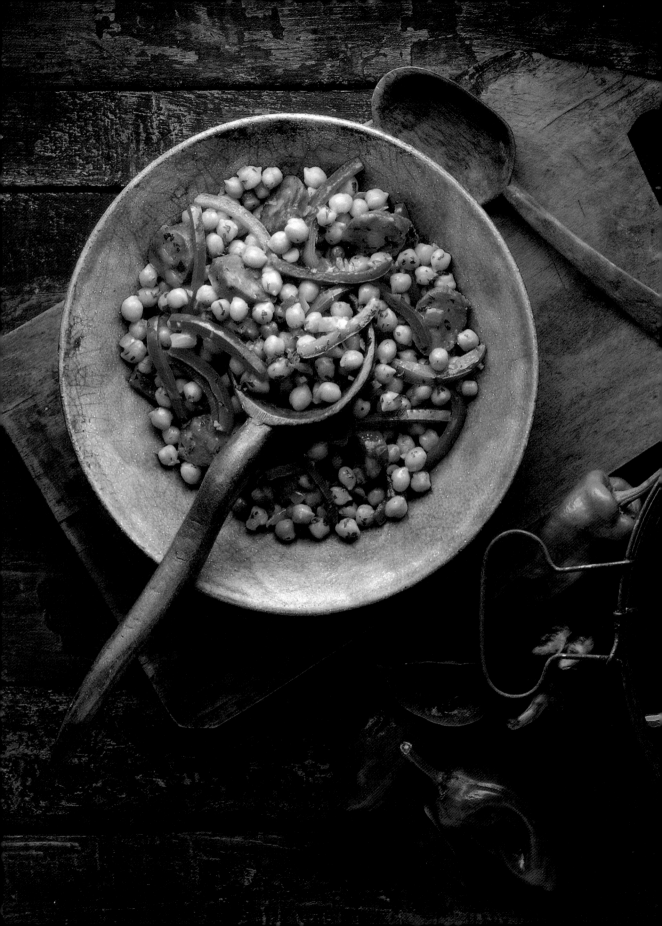

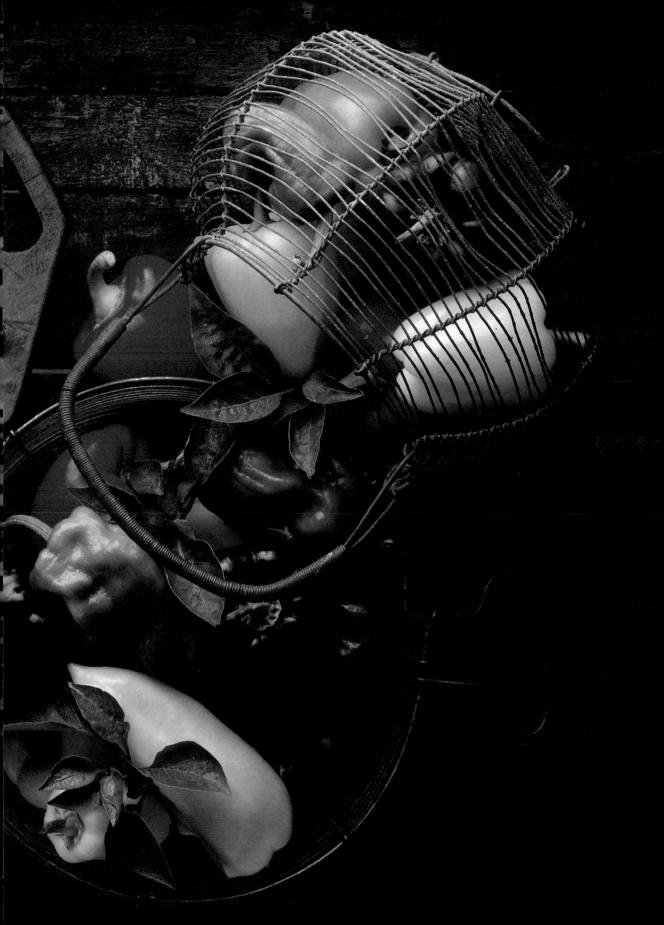

Tuna and Frisée Salad
with Grilled Red Dressing

This salad was inspired by a Catalan dish called Xato, though I've simplified and twiddled with it so much that it can lay no claims to being the original. Nonetheless, it tastes very good with its smoky dressing made from grilled peppers, chillies, garlic and tomato. A word of warning, however – don't toss the salad until after everyone has seen it. The thick dressing may taste good, but it makes the salad look a bit gungy.

For this recipe, you will need thick-fleshed chillies as they have to be grilled and skinned. Fresno and Jalapeno chillies are ideal and luckily they are readily available. The conical fresh green chillies, usually imported from Kenya, with broad shoulders tapering quickly to a point, that are sold in most supermarkets will be either Fresno or Jalapeno.

SERVES 4

½ a head of frisée lettuce
1 × 200-g (7-oz) tin tuna, drained and flaked

2 hard-boiled eggs, quartered
4 anchovy fillets, halved lengthwise

For the dressing

1 red pepper
1 Fresno *or* Jalapeno green chilli
3 cloves garlic
225 g (8 oz) tomatoes

1 tablespoon red wine vinegar
1 teaspoon sugar
Salt
6 tablespoons extra virgin olive oil

To make the dressing, grill the red pepper and chilli close to the heat, turning occasionally, until skins are blackened and blistered. Drop into a plastic bag, knot the ends and leave until cool enough to handle. Meanwhile, thread the garlic cloves onto a skewer and grill close to the heat until charred and softened. Grill the tomatoes until soft.

Skin the pepper, chilli and tomatoes. Peel the garlic. Liquidize or process pepper, chilli, tomato and garlic with the vinegar, sugar and a little salt. Keep the motor running and gradually trickle in the olive oil. Taste and adjust seasoning.

Pour dressing into a salad bowl. Wash and dry the frisée lettuce, then tear into manageable pieces. Arrange over the dressing and scatter with the tuna. Arrange eggs and anchovy fillets on top. Toss at the table.

Peppers Stuffed with Crab and Pasta

Peppers are tailor-made containers for stuffings, and they take well to all kinds of fillings. In this recipe, I've packed them full of pasta and crab (fresh not frozen, please). If you can't find any of the tiddly pasta shapes that are meant for soup, you can always break up dry spaghetti instead.

When I'm preparing peppers for stuffing, I usually blanch them briefly first. This speeds up the final baking process and, I think, improves their flavour and texture. You can skip this bit if you wish, and increase their time in the oven by 15 mintues or so, but check that they are not drying out – add a little more water and cover with foil if necessary.

SERVES 4 as a first course, 2 as a main course

4 red *and/or* green peppers
1 tablespoon olive oil

For the filling

75 g (3 oz) small pasta shapes
(e.g. stelline)
2 cloves garlic, peeled and chopped
2 tablespoons olive oil
175 g (6 oz) crab meat, half brown, half white, flaked
225 g (8 oz) tomatoes, skinned, de-seeded and diced

4 spring onions, thinly sliced
1 tablespoon finely chopped fresh parsley
1 teaspoon Dijon mustard
½ tablespoon white wine vinegar
Salt and freshly ground black pepper

Cook the pasta in salted boiling water for 3 minutes until almost, but not quite *al dente*. Drain well. Cook the garlic in a small pan in a little of the oil over a low heat, until lightly coloured. Mix with the pasta, remaining oil and all the remaining filling ingredients. Taste and adjust seasoning.

Pre-heat the oven to gas mark 5, 375°F (190°C). Bring a large pan of lightly salted water to the boil and drop the whole peppers into it. Bring back to the boil and simmer for 5 minutes. Drain, then slice off the tops to form lids, and clean out the seeds. Fill the peppers with the pasta and crab mixture and stand in a close-fitting oiled shallow ovenproof dish, replacing lids on the filled peppers. Drizzle over the tablespoon of olive oil, and spoon 5 tablespoons of water around them. Bake for 30–40 minutes until tender. Serve hot, warm or cold.

Baked Monkfish with Coriander and Red Peppers

This recipe brings together a whole host of my favourite ingredients: grilled red peppers, firm monkfish, coriander, garlic, soy sauce and olive oil. Bliss. Monkfish isn't cheap, alas, so it's a special-occasion-only dish, but what a treat it is.

SERVES 4

2 red peppers
1 × 750 g–1 kg (1½–2 lb) monkfish tail
8 spring onions, cut into 5-cm (2-inch) lengths
2 tablespoons roughly chopped fresh coriander

2 cloves garlic, finely chopped
1 tablespoon dark soy sauce
Juice of ½ lemon
5 tablespoons olive oil
Salt and freshly ground black pepper

Quarter the red peppers and grill, skin-side up, as close as possible to the heat, until they are blackened and blistered all over. Drop into a plastic bag, knot the end, and leave until cool enough to handle whilst you get on with organizing the rest of the dish.

Pre-heat the oven to gas mark 5, 375°F (190°C). Pull off the thin membrane covering the monkfish tail if the fishmonger hasn't already done it. Place the tail in an oiled ovenproof dish. Scatter the spring onions, coriander and garlic around and over the fish. Return to the peppers, and strip off the blackened skins. Cut into strips and scatter over the fish, along with any juice from the peppers. Pour 4 tablespoons water around the fish, then trickle the soy sauce, lemon juice and olive oil evenly over it. Season lightly with salt and pepper.

Roast the fish, uncovered, for 25–30 minutes, basting occasionally with its own juices, until cooked through. Serve immediately.

Pisto

Julian Diment-Castillo and his brother Robert are both students at Bristol University. They share a flat tucked away at the top of a house. Their mother is Spanish and runs three of the best tapas bars in London. Every summer the family heads off to their home near Valencia, bringing back ample supplies of local olive oil when they return. Julian is a keen cook, though restricted by the paucity of the student grant. He loves making Spanish food and this dish is one that he turns to often. It's quick and easy to prepare and, what's more, tastes delicious. The traditional way of eating it is to place the dish in the middle of the table and let everyone dig in, using plenty of good bread to mop the dish clean.

SERVES 4 as a first course, 2 as a main course

3 tablespoons olive oil
1 onion, roughly chopped
2 cloves garlic, peeled and chopped
1 red pepper, de-seeded and cut roughly
    into 2.5-cm (1-inch) squares
1 green pepper, de-seeded and cut
    roughly into 2.5-cm (1-inch) squares

1 yellow pepper (or a second red one),
    de-seeded and cut roughly into
    2.5-cm (1-inch) squares
1 × 400 g (14 oz) tin tomatoes
½ teaspoon dried mixed herbs *or* 1
    tablespoon chopped fresh parsley
Salt and freshly ground black pepper
2 eggs

Pre-heat the oven to gas mark 5, 375°F (190°C).

Warm the oil in a frying-pan and add the onion and garlic. Cook gently for about 3 minutes. Add the peppers and continue cooking over a gentle heat until the peppers are tender, without letting them brown. Add the tomatoes, herbs, salt and pepper. Simmer for about 15 minutes, breaking up the tomatoes with a spoon, until the peppers are bathed in a thick tomato sauce.

Quickly pour the mixture into an ovenproof dish and carefully break the eggs on top of it. Bake for about 10 minutes until the egg whites are just set. Serve immediately with lots of good bread to mop up the juices.

SALADS

Lettuces • Rocket, Sorrel and Purslane

Chicory and Radicchio

Watercress • Radishes

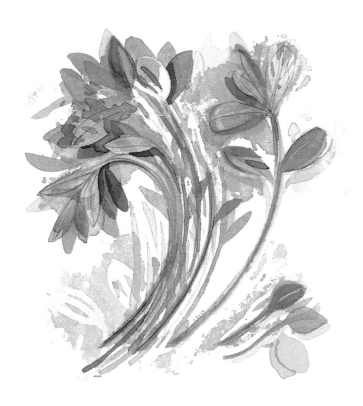

Lettuces

To say that Frances Smith grows lettuces is like saying that the Queen has a penny or two to rub together. Frances grows every type of salad leaf imaginable and chefs troop up from miles away to pick and choose greenery for the fanciest of designer salads. Her astounding collection has been built up over many years. Whenever she journeys abroad, she makes a beeline for seed shops in search of new varieties to try out.

Amongst the more familiar lettuces that she picks as saladings when young and delicate, there are stranger relations: bronzed, crinkled, curved, spikey, bitter, hot and sweet leaves to give green salads complex and intriguing blends of flavours. Frances has firm ideas about how to compose a salad. She starts with a base of lettuce, at least one mild one and perhaps a bitter one too, for bulk. Next she adds something for flavour – maybe peppery rocket or hot Fordhook mustard leaves. Third is an element for texture, velvety green lambs lettuce, or more assertive sprouted shoots or mangetout peas, and finally something pretty, frivolous and unusual – golden oregano, nasturtium flowers, or twining green pea tendrils.

Lettuces proper fall into one of two main groups: headed lettuces and loose non-hearting lettuces. Headed lettuces include the butterhead types, which have floppy, soft leaves and in my opinion are hardly worth bothering with, and the much more satisfying crispheads, such as Webb's Wonder (one of the best) and the tasteless but crunchy iceberg. Cos lettuce, also headed, is the most delicious of all lettuces. Little Gem lettuces are sometimes described as semi-cos for their upright nature and crisp pale yellow heart.

Many of the fashionably pretty lettuces of the eighties are non-hearting. Bronzed and green oak leaf, for example, and frilly lollo rosso and lollo biondo. In flavour, they can be on the dull side, but they look ravishing. Curly endives or frisée, are not really lettuces at all – their bitter edge betrays their membership of the chicory clan.

Preparing Salad Leaves

Whether you use a singleton or a mixture of salad leaves, the rules of salad making are straightforward, though often sadly neglected. Frances Smith advises salad growers to pick leaves only as required, laying them gently in a basket, or slipping them into small plastic bags to carry them back to the kitchen. From then on the same rules apply to home-grown and shop bought salads. The first thing to do is to wash them, rinsing and swishing the leaves around carefully in a large bowl of water to avoid bruising. On a hot day leave them in the water for an hour or two to crisp up. Then drain and dry them, ready for use.

Washed lettuce leaves should be used as soon as possible, though they can be kept crisp in a plastic bag in the fridge, moistened with a few drops of water, for several hours. Make sure that they are dry before you use them – a damp salad is a damp squib. If necessary, pat the leaves dry, lightly and lovingly, in a clean tea towel or kitchen paper, or whizz them briefly in a salad spinner.

Always make salad dressings with the best quality oils and vinegars that you can afford. It should not be so sharp that your mouth puckers when you taste it. Never toss the salad until it is on the table and ready to serve. Leaves doused in vinaigrette droop and darken with brutal speed. And finally, don't overdo the dressing – a light coating is all that is required.

Though the greatest charm of lettuces lies in the salad bowl, they can be cooked as well. Tight hearted lettuces like Little Gem are very good braised and hold their shape tolerably well. In soups lettuce adds a sweet unidentifiable smoothness – add it shredded with the rest of the vegetables.

Basic Vinaigrette

Please don't waste your money on bottles of ready-made French dressing. They are ridiculously expensive and not terribly good either. Making a proper vinaigrette or French dressing is child's play. Of course, you'll have to invest in a decent bottle of oil, either extra virgin olive oil or plainer groundnut oil, and another of wine vinegar, but they can be used for other things too.

Any left-over vinaigrette will keep in a screwtop jar in the fridge for several weeks. In fact, I usually make double or treble quantities, so that there's plenty left to use at a moment's notice.

ENOUGH FOR a generous 6-person salad

1 tablespoon wine vinegar
½ teaspoon Dijon mustard (*optional*)

Salt and freshly ground black pepper
4–5 tablespoons olive oil
or groundnut oil

In a salad bowl, mix the vinegar with the mustard, salt and pepper. Whisk in the oil, a tablespoon at a time. After the fourth spoonful, taste – if it is on the sharp side, whisk in the last spoonful of oil and more if necessary. Adjust seasonings.

Alternatively put all ingredients into a screw-top jar, close tightly and shake to mix. Taste and adjust seasoning or add more oil, as necessary.

Anchovy Dressing

This is a powerfully flavoured dressing so save it to use on robust salads. I love it with slightly bitter frisée and rocket, with a scattering of diced tomato.

ENOUGH FOR a generous 6-person salad

4 anchovy fillets, chopped
1 small clove garlic, peeled
1 tablespoon sherry vinegar
    or red wine vinegar

Freshly ground black pepper
4–5 tablespoons olive oil

In a mortar or small bowl pound the chopped anchovy fillets and garlic to a paste. Add the vinegar and pound and mix until creamy. Season with plenty of pepper and beat in the oil a tablespoon at a time. Taste and adjust seasonings adding more oil if needed.

Serve with a salad of frisée, and finely chopped tomato.

Green Leaf Salad with Walnuts

Even supermarkets now sell the rarer nut oils, and a jolly good thing too. A vinaigrette made with nut oil and a scattering of matching toasted nuts gives a simple salad a major lift. Walnuts and walnut oil are excellent, but you might also try toasted hazelnuts or pine kernels with hazelnut oil.

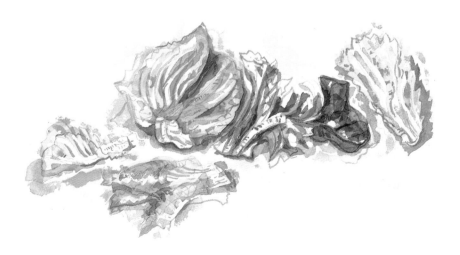

SERVES 4

25 g (1 oz) walnut pieces
Selection of salad leaves (e.g. cos, frisée,
    radicchio, batavia, lollo rosso)

For the dressing

1 tablespoon red wine vinegar
½–1 clove garlic, peeled and crushed
    (*optional*)
Salt and freshly ground black pepper

Pinch of sugar
3 tablespoons walnut oil and
    2 tablespoons sunflower
    or groundnut oil

Pre-heat the oven to gas mark 6–8, 400–450°F (200–230°C).

Spread the walnut pieces out on a baking sheet and cook for 5–10 minutes, shaking tray occasionally, until the walnuts are patched with dark brown. Tip into a wire sieve and shake to dislodge any papery flakes of skin. Cool.

Wash and dry the salad leaves. Store in a knotted plastic bag in the bottom of the fridge, until needed. Either put all dressing ingredients in a screwtop jar and shake well to mix, or whisk the vinegar with the garlic, salt, pepper and sugar and then gradually whisk in the oil. Taste and adjust seasonings.

Just before serving shake the dressing, and pour about half of it (save the rest for another salad) into a salad bowl. Cross salad servers in the bowl, and arrange the leaves on top. Scatter with the walnuts and toss at table.

Braised Lettuce with Mushroom and Bacon

Lettuce is only for salads . . . or is it? Not necessarily. Tightly furled dense Little Gem lettuces or hearts of other salads survive cooking extremely well, softening down but not dissolving away. Braised with mushrooms and bacon they make a delicious side dish to any main course.

SERVES 4

4 Little Gem lettuces
100 g (4 oz) unsmoked back bacon, in
    one piece *or* thick cut
25 g (1 oz) butter
1 onion, chopped

225 g (8 oz) button mushrooms,
    quartered
1 sprig of fresh thyme
1 tablespoon chopped fresh parsley
1 teaspoon sugar
Salt and freshly ground black pepper

Remove and discard any damaged outer leaves of the lettuces. Then cut the whole lettuces in half lengthwise and rinse well. Drain thoroughly. Dice the bacon into 5-mm (¼-inch) cubes.

Melt the butter in a saucepan large enough to take all the lettuce halves in a tight single layer. Add the bacon, onion, mushrooms, thyme and parsley, give them a quick stir, and then snuggle in the lettuces. Sprinkle with sugar, salt and pepper. Cover tightly and cook over a very gentle heat for 15 minutes, occasionally turning and basting the lettuces. Remove the lid and simmer for a further 5 minutes, until the lettuces are tender.

If there is still an ocean of liquid in the pan, scoop out the lettuces, bacon and mushrooms on to a serving dish, keep them warm and boil the pan juices hard until reduced by a third or so. Pour over the lettuces and serve.

Wilted Salad with Goat's Cheese and Sun-dried Tomatoes

Grilled goat's cheese served with salad has become a standard first course in chic cafés and brasseries. This salad goes one step further, by grilling the entire salad to produce a sensational combination of warm and cool, melting cheese and buttery crisp pinenuts, bitter and sweet leaves.

SERVES 4

½ head of radicchio, leaves separated and roughly torn up
1 handful of rocket leaves
8 leaves cos *or* Webb's lettuce, roughly torn up

For the dressing
2 tablespoons olive oil
½ tablespoon balsamic, sherry *or* red wine vinegar
Salt and freshly ground black pepper

100 g (4 oz) goat's cheese, rind removed, diced
6 pieces of sun-dried tomato, cut into thin strips
15 g (½ oz) pine kernels, lightly toasted

First make the dressing. Whisk the oil into the vinegar a spoonful at a time. Season with salt and pepper.

Mix the salad leaves. Just before serving, toss salad leaves in a bowl with dressing so that they are evenly coated. Spread them out in a 30-cm (12-inch) gratin dish and scatter over cheese, tomatoes and pine kernels. Whizz under a pre-heated grill for 3–4 minutes, until the salad leaves are wilting and goat's cheese is beginning to soften. Serve immediately.

Warm Chorizo (or Bacon) and Frisée Salad

When fried to a sizzling brown, spicy Spanish chorizo sausage gives off a fairly copious amount of fat. Add garlic and a generous splash of vinegar and you can create a sensational dressing for a substantial salad. I serve this both as a main course and as a starter but, either way, friends always clear their plates and beg for seconds.

If you can't get chorizo, buy a slab of bacon and use that instead.

SERVES 6 as a first course, 4 as a main course

225–275 g (8–10 oz) chorizo sausage
  or slab bacon
Generous bowlful of frisée *or* dandelion
  leaves *or* a mixture of robust leaves
3 tablespoons extra virgin olive oil

1–2 cloves garlic, peeled and chopped
1 tablespoon red wine vinegar
Salt and freshly ground black pepper
6 spring onions, sliced

Skin the chorizo, if using, and cut into slices about 5 mm (¼ inch) thick. If using bacon, cut into batons, about 2.5 cm (1 inch) long by a generous 5 mm (¼ inch) thick and wide. Pick over and wash the salad leaves, and dry thoroughly. Place in a large salad bowl.

Heat the oil in a wide frying-pan over a generous heat, and add the chorizo or bacon. Fry for about 1 minute and then add the garlic. Fry until chorizo (or bacon) is browned.

Draw off the heat, and let it stand for about 15 seconds or so, then add the vinegar, stir and quickly pour over the salad. Add salt and pepper, toss and finally scatter with spring onions. Serve immediately.

Caesar Salad

There are many recipes for this most famous of salads, invented in the 1920s by Caesar Cardini at his restaurant in Tijuana, Mexico. The original didn't include anchovies, but they often creep in none the less. The final preparation (which I've simplified a little) can be done discreetly in the kitchen, or more dramatically at the dinner table. If you choose to perform publicly, make sure you have a very large bowl, so that you don't shower your audience with lettuce.

SERVES 6

2 cos lettuces
3 slices stale white bread, crusts removed, cut into 1-cm (½-inch)
  cubes
3 cloves garlic
160 ml (5 fl oz) extra virgin olive oil
2 eggs

½ tin anchovy fillets, finely chopped
  or ½ teaspoon Worcestershire
  sauce
Juice of 1 lemon
Salt and freshly ground black pepper
25 g (1 oz) freshly grated Parmesan
  cheese

IN ADVANCE: Wash and dry the lettuce well. Store in the fridge in a plastic bag until needed. Fry the cubes of bread with the garlic in 5 tablespoons of the olive oil, until golden and crisp. Drain the croûtons on kitchen paper. Put the eggs into a pan, cover with water, and bring to the boil. Boil for 1 minute, then drain and run under the cold tap.

AT THE LAST MINUTE: Tear the lettuce up into manageable pieces and place in a large salad bowl. Pour over 6 tablespoons of olive oil and toss to coat each leaf. Add anchovies or Worcestershire sauce, croûtons, lemon juice, pepper and a little salt. Toss. Finally break in the eggs, taking care not to get specks of shell into the salad, and scatter with the Parmesan. Toss or turn again to mix evenly. Now, with all the work done, you can serve it.

OVERLEAF *Caesar Salad*

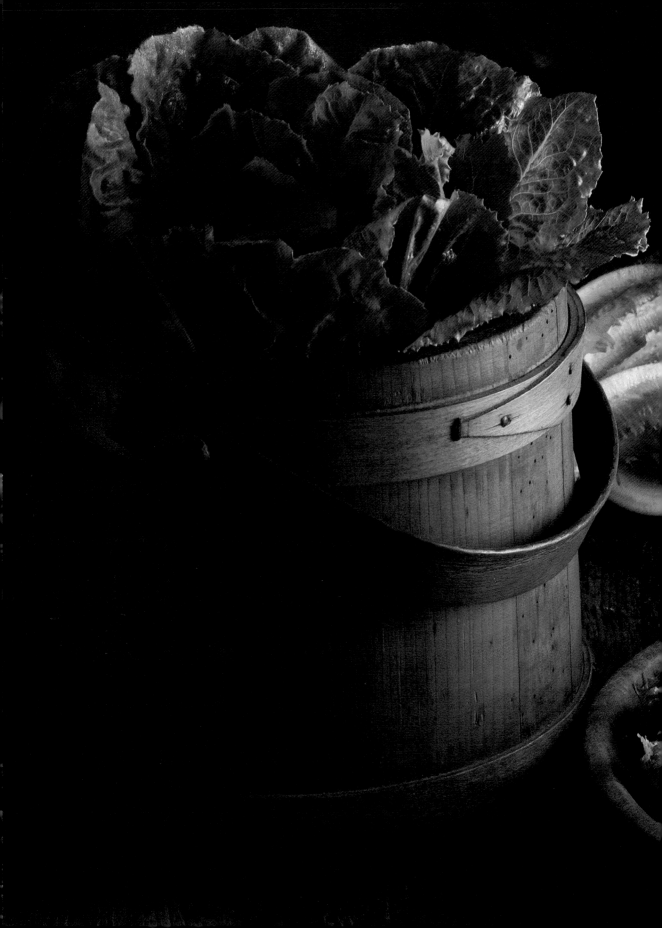

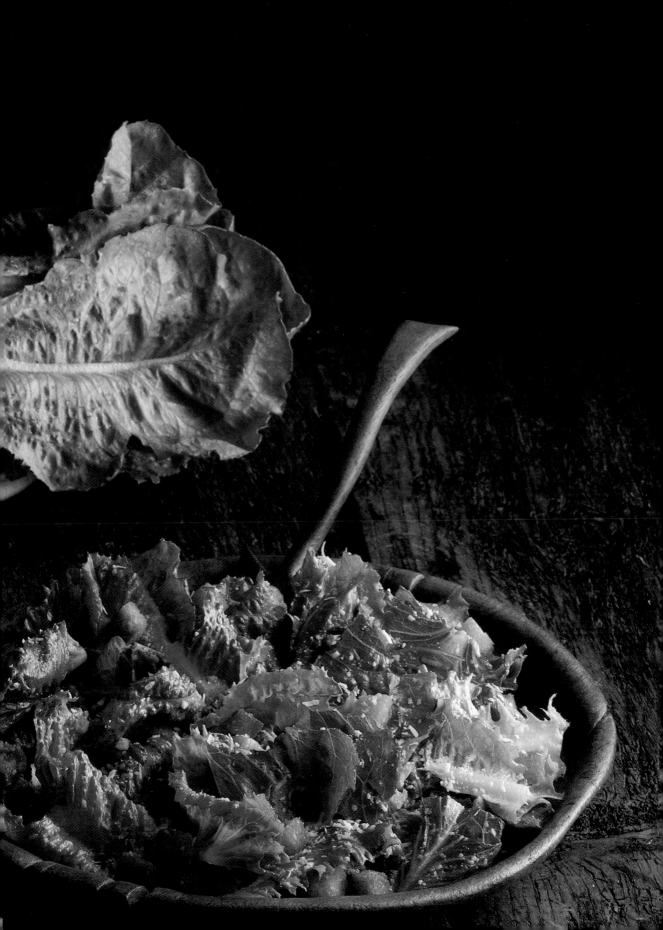

Rocket, Sorrel and Purslane

In 1664 John Evelyn listed 35 plants in his salad calendar. Besides lettuces, there were nasturtiums, radish leaves, a handful of herbs, shallots and onion. Rocket, sorrel and purslane had their place in the scheme as well. All three were raised in British gardens for centuries, and then all three fell out of favour and disappeared. Why, one wonders, when they grow so easily and have such distinctive and welcome flavours? There is no good reason for the whims of fashion, but at least fashion is bringing them back again. Creeping in first came rocket, then sorrel and lastly, more slowly and cautiously, purslane.

Rocket has never lost its status in Italy, where it is known as arugula or rucola or in Greece and Cyprus where the name is rokka. It has a wonderful, peppery green taste that can become quite addictive. Small leaves, that look a little like curvaceous young dandelion greens, are sometimes sold as 'roquette', which strikes me as pretty silly when there is a perfectly good English name. In my local Greek-Cypriot greengrocers, they sell big bunches of coarser large-leafed rocket which is ideal for cooking.

I always think of sorrel as more of a French plant. We used to nibble at the lemony leaves as children in France – there was always a plant in every garden. It grows just as sturdily and happily here. Though the raw leaves, torn into shreds, add a nice sharp contrast in mixed green salads, I tend to reserve French sorrel for cooking. Buckler Leaf sorrel is a variety with small shield-shaped leaves and a less mouth-puckering acidity, which makes it a better bet for salads.

Purslane is the most outlandish of the trio with fleshy green leaves which vary deeply in flavour according to size and variety. It grows wild in many areas of the Mediterranean; in Nice it is one of a quartet of wild herbs known as refrescat, simmered in soups to which it gives a special freshness and smoothness. Claytonia, which may also be called Winter Purslane or Miner's Lettuce, is a close relative of purslane. It is enchantingly coquettish with tiny white flowers that grow up through the leaf like a spring posy. Claytonia doesn't have a great deal of taste, to be honest, but it is worth growing because it looks so lovely perched on a salad, or as a decorative aside on a dinner plate.

Preparing Rocket, Sorrel and Purslane

Prepare rocket as you would any salad leaf, washing and drying it carefully to avoid unnecessary bruising. A handful of young rocket leaves in a green salad adds incomparable vigour, but I like it so much that I often use it as a salad on its own. And it makes superb sandwiches – clamped with a few shavings of Parmesan between two pieces of bread moistened with olive oil and a rub of garlic. In Italy it is used to make soups and may also be dished up on hot pasta, limpened only by the heat of the pasta itself.

Coarser mature rocket is sturdy enough (and cheap enough) to withstand cooking. Thrown into boiling water, bought back to the boil, and then drained, large-leafed rocket makes an excellent side-dish to serve with grilled meats or fish, or it can be bathed with olive oil and lemon juice and left to cool for a salad.

The most common way to cook sorrel is by turning it into a purée to use in sauces to partner fish and in soup and egg dishes. Wash the leaves carefully, then snip off the tough green stems. Pile leaves up four or five at a time and shred finely, then stew briefly in butter or oil until the shreds melt down to a dark green mass. The purée freezes well – handy if you have a surfeit of leaves to deal with. Shredded sorrel leaves can also be added discretely to salads for sharpness, or thrown straight into the saucepan with the other vegetables when making soup.

Small-leaved purslane with red stalks has a fresh, nutty and cool flavour which makes it a lovely salad leaf. Larger-leafed purslane with green stalks, the only kind I've found for sale commercially (in Greek-Cypriot and Middle Eastern food shops), can be astringent, so should be chopped and mixed in with plenty of other salad ingredients when it is to be eaten raw, or blanched or cooked briefly. Purslane is the essential ingredient in the marvellous Middle Eastern salad, fatoush (see p. 189), but it is also good in omelettes and soups amongst other things.

OVERLEAF *Fusilli with Smoked Trout, Rocket and Basil*

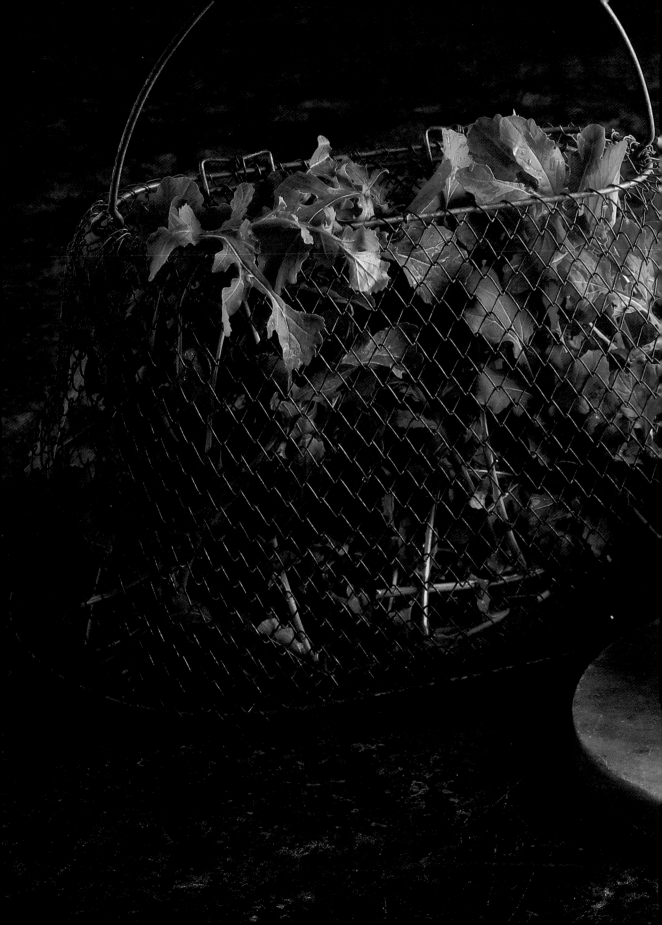

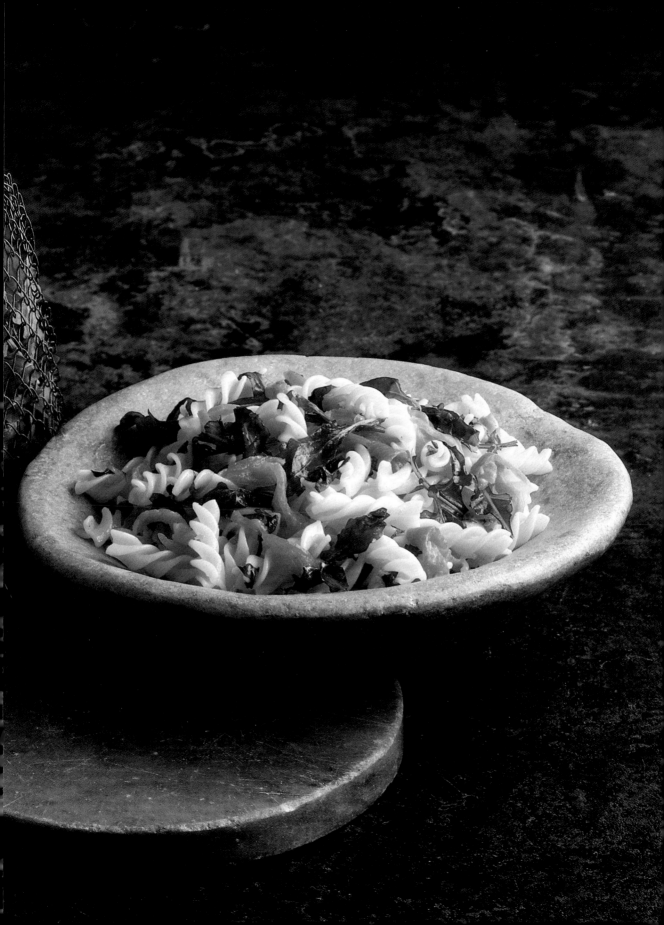

Fusilli with Smoked Trout, Rocket and Basil

This dish takes just minutes to make – the rocket, basil and smoked fish cooking instantly in the heat of the pasta.

SERVES 4

1 handful of rocket leaves
400 g (14 oz) fusilli *or* other pasta shapes
6 tablespoons olive oil
Juice of ½ lemon
2 cloves garlic, peeled and crushed

Salt and freshly ground black pepper
12 large fresh basil leaves, shredded
175 g (6 oz) sliced smoked trout, cut
    into short thin strips

If the rocket leaves are fairly large, tear them up roughly. If they are tiny, 5 cm (2 inches) or so in length, tear or snip them in half. Prepare all the remaining ingredients.

Cook the fusilli in a large pan of lightly salted water until just *al dente*. Drain well and return to the pan, set over a low heat. Toss in the olive oil, lemon juice, garlic, a little salt and plenty of pepper. Stir for a couple of seconds, then add the rocket and basil and toss again to mix evenly. Draw off the heat and finally toss in the trout. Serve immediately.

Pancoto con Rucola e Patate
[Rocket and Potato Soup]

This is a peasant soup from Apulia, the heel of Italy. Filling and thick with potatoes and bread, it's the peppery rocket and the final touch of garlic fried in olive oil that hoists it into the realms of truly satisfying food. When made with water it's good, but it's even better with a good stock.

SERVES 4

1 kg (2 lb) potatoes, peeled and diced
Salt
900 ml (1½ pints) water *or* light chicken
    stock *or* water left over from
    cooking vegetables
75 g (3 oz) rocket leaves, roughly
    chopped

Cayenne pepper
4 thick slices of stale bread (about
    100 g, 4 oz)
5 tablespoons olive oil
3 cloves garlic, peeled and sliced

Put the potatoes into a saucepan with the water or stock, and salt. Bring to the boil and simmer for 10 minutes. Add the rocket and continue cooking for 15 minutes. Taste and add more salt if needed and a shake of cayenne pepper. Draw off the heat, add the bread, and leave to stand, covered, for 10 minutes.

While the soup is standing, fry the garlic in the olive oil until golden brown. Pour over the soup, dust lightly with a little more cayenne, and serve, stirring garlicky oil into the soup as you spoon it into bowls.

Fattoush

Visiting salad-grower Frances Smith gave me the perfect opportunity to try out a salad I'd longed to make. Fattoush is a Middle Eastern salad and, though I'd made approximations of it before, this was the first time I'd made it with purslane, the essential ingredient. It makes a huge difference to the flavour, though to be honest I'd always enjoyed it without.

SERVES 6–8

1 cucumber, diced
Salt and freshly ground black pepper
1 pitta bread
Juice of 1 lemon
4 tomatoes, de-seeded and diced
6 spring onions
    or 1 medium red onion, chopped

Leaves of 1 small bunch of purslane,
    chopped if large
4 tablespoons chopped fresh parsley
2 tablespoons chopped fresh mint
2 tablespoons chopped fresh coriander
2 cloves garlic, peeled and crushed
6–7 tablespoons olive oil

Spread the cucumber dice out in a colander and sprinkle lightly with salt. Leave for 30 minutes to drain. Rinse and dry on kitchen paper.

Split open the pitta bread and toast with the opened side to the heat, until browned and crisp. Break up into small pieces and place in a salad bowl. Sprinkle with about a third of the lemon juice. Now add all the remaining ingredients including the cucumber. Turn with your hands to mix. Taste and adjust seasoning, adding more lemon juice if needed.

Cooked Purslane

If the purslane leaves are large and astringent, drop them into a pan of lightly salted boiling water. Bring back to the boil and drain immediately. Drain well and dress with butter, salt and freshly ground black pepper, to serve hot, or with olive oil, a squeeze of lemon, salt and freshly ground black pepper to serve cold.

To make a more robust cold cooked purslane salad, add strips of grilled red pepper, quartered cherry tomatoes, or sprinkle with chopped hard-boiled egg and fresh parsley, and perhaps some olives. Or add cubes of feta.

Purslane Omelette

A simple way to use purslane, but particularly good when the leaves have grown too large and astringent to eat raw.

SERVES 1

1 handful of purslane
Generous knob of butter
2–3 eggs, beaten
Salt and freshly ground black pepper

If the purslane leaves are large, chop the leaves and discard the tough stalks. If they are small and tender, then chop the whole lot roughly. Heat the butter in an omelette pan and add the purslane. Cook for a few minutes until just tender. Meanwhile, season the eggs generously with salt and pepper. Pour over the purslane, stir lightly and cook as for a normal omelette.

Sorrel Omelette

Follow the recipe for Purslane omelette above, using shredded sorrel, cooked for just a few brief seconds before pouring in the eggs and stirring. Then continue as usual.

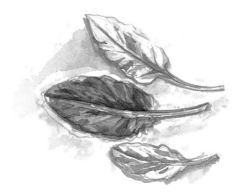

Sorrel Sauce

Sorrel is the basis for one of the classic sauces for fish (though I like it with chicken and eggs as well). Tart and creamy it adds a note of luxury. Stir any juices that seep out as the fish cooks into the sauce just before serving. For a lighter sauce, reduce the amount of cream and replace it with fish stock.

SERVES 4
2 handfuls of sorrel
25 g (1 oz) butter
150 ml (5 fl oz) double cream
Juices from cooking fish *or* a splash of
    fish stock (*optional*)
Salt and freshly ground black pepper

Snip off the stems of the sorrel leaves and discard. Shred the leaves finely. Heat the butter in a pan, and add the sorrel. Stir over a moderate heat until the sorrel dissolves to a rough purée. Stir in the cream and any cooking juices or a splash of fish stock if using. Return to the heat and cook for a few minutes. Serve hot.

Chicory and Radicchio

There was a time when tapering, ivory digits of chicory were sold swaddled in dark blue waxed paper to protect them from the light. It was a sound practice, for darkness is as essential to chicory as sunlight is to a sunflower. Belgian or Witloof chicory, to give it its full name, is 'forced' from fully formed roots, their leaves and tips trimmed off before they are planted, huddling close together in the dark. Within four to five weeks, the blanched 'chicons' will be thrusting up, six inches or so long, pale ghostly white with bands of yellow edging the tips of the leaves.

Forcing tames and refines the flavour, pushing out the intense natural bitterness so that the chicory has just a pleasing mild bitter edge and is tender and juicy. Exposed to light for any length of time, even after they have been harvested, the pale yellow edging changes to green and the bitterness begins to seep back in.

Good chicory is firm and unblemished with yellow rather than green or browning edges to the leaves. The chicons should be tightly packed, tapering neatly to a point. Sometimes you may have no choice but to buy ones with some bruising on the outer leaves. As long as the damage is not extensive, they can be stripped off. Store chicory in brown paper in the bottom of the fridge, where it will keep for four or five days.

There is also a red form of forced chicory, which tastes similar and looks very pretty, but not all forms of chicory are forced. Sugar loaf chicory looks a little like cos lettuce and is self-blanching. The green outer leaves add a delicious bitter note to salads, but their main job is to hide the heart from the light leaving it more like forced chicory in taste. Radicchio is red, unforced chicory, that grows green until the cold weather sets in, triggering the transformation to dark purple red streaked with white.

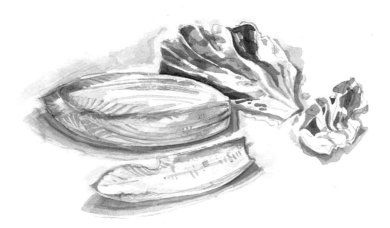

Preparing Chicory and Radicchio

Wash chicons briefly and dry, then trim the base. Some cooks whittle a small cone out of the base which is supposed to reduce the bitterness, but I've never found that it makes any noticeable difference.

Raw chicory, sliced about 5 mm (¼ inch) thick is lovely in salads and especially welcome in winter. The individual leaves can be separated out and used with dips of one sort or another. In France you are much more likely to come across cooked chicory than raw. Heat gives it a completely different nature, enhancing the bitterness though never to the degree that it becomes unpleasant. The chicons can simply be simmered (add the juice of half a lemon and a teaspoon of sugar to the water) or steamed until tender but still with a slight firmness at the centre. They need thorough draining to expel all the water that gathers amongst the leaves. It is a good idea to squeeze them gently with your hands, working from base down to the tip. The chicory will taste ten times better if you undercook it slightly, squeeze out the water, then fry it gently in butter until patched with brown. A hint of sweetness suits chicory well, as does orange juice. Both are used in the recipes that follow.

As with chicory, brown-edged leaves are a bad sign in radicchio. The tight balls of red should be firm and glowing. For salads ease off as many leaves as you need and shred them thickly so that there will be streaks of magenta running through the rest of the greenery. Whole leaves, as long as they are not floppy, can be used as little cups for finely diced salads coated in vinaigrette, or sturdier affairs with flaked tinned tuna, or shredded cooked chicken bound with mayonnaise.

Cooked radicchio is as good as chicory in its own way, though the red turns a murky brown which is a disappointment. Whole leaves can be floured, egged, crumbed and deep-fried as an hors d'oeuvre. Or you could quarter the heads, brush them with oil and grill until semi-tender. Season with salt, pepper, lemon juice or a few drops of balsamic or sherry vinegar. Fried shredded radicchi makes an expectedly interesting accompaniment to fish or a meaty steak.

Endivio con Rocfort
[Chicory with Roquefort]

Chicory with a blue cheese dressing is a common hors d'œuvre in the small restaurants of Barcelona. There they may use French Roquefort, or a Spanish blue cheese called Cabrales which has a similar flavour.

Sᴇʀᴠᴇꜱ 4–6

3 heads of chicory

For the dressing

40 g (1½ oz) Roquefort *or* Cabrales
5 tablespoons mayonnaise
2–3 tablespoons milk

Squeeze of lemon
2 tablespoons chopped fresh parsley
Cayenne pepper

Either quarter the heads of chicory lengthwise, or separate into individual leaves. Arrange on a serving plate, and cover.

Mash the cheese to a paste, and then beat in the mayonnaise, followed by the milk. Stir in the lemon juice, parsley and cayenne pepper. Taste and adjust seasonings, adding more lemon juice or cayenne if you think it needs it. Spoon over the quartered chicory. If you've separated out the leaves, place a spoonful of dressing in the curve of each leaf at the widest end. Serve.

Chicory, Watercress and Orange Salad

I always think of this as a Christmas salad, though there's no good reason not to make it at any time of the year. It's just that it goes particularly well with cold ham and turkey.

Sᴇʀᴠᴇꜱ 6–8

2 bunches of watercress
3 heads of chicory, sliced into rounds
2 oranges, peeled and cut into chunks
40 g (1½ oz) walnut pieces

For the dressing

1 tablespoon sherry vinegar *or* red wine
    vinegar
Pinch of sugar
Salt and freshly ground black pepper

5 tablespoons extra virgin olive oil
    or 3 tablespoons walnut oil and
    2 tablespoons sunflower oil

Either put all the dressing ingredients in a screwtop jar and shake well to mix, or whisk the vinegar with the sugar, salt and pepper and then gradually whisk in the oil(s). Taste and adjust seasonings and pour into a salad bowl, and cross salad servers in the bowl over the dressing.

Wash and pick over the watercress and remove any damaged leaves. Tear into small pieces. Place in the bowl over the servers. Scatter chicory, orange and walnuts over the top. Toss at the table.

Red Mullet with Chicory and Orange

With its strong, gamey taste, red mullet is a fish that can carry the equally strong, bitter flavour of chicory in easy partnership. The chicory is cooked down to a moist sweet-bitter citrussy mass and served as an essential element with the fish.

SERVES 2

½ large orange
15 g (½ oz) butter
1 tablespoon finely chopped onion
2 heads of chicory, sliced 5 mm (¼ inch) thick
1 tablespoon lemon juice

1 teaspoon sugar
2 × 175–225 g (6–8 oz) red mullet scaled and cleaned
Salt and freshly ground black pepper
Olive oil for brushing
A little chopped fresh parsley to garnish

Pare 4 wide strips of zest off the half orange, and cut into thin shreds. Blanch in boiling water for 2 minutes. Drain and set aside. Squeeze the juice from the orange and set aside.

Melt the butter in a small saucepan over a fairly low heat. Add the onion and cook gently until tender, without browning. Add the chicory and continue cooking, stirring, for a further 2 minutes or so. Mix in the orange juice, lemon juice, and sugar. Simmer, stirring occasionally, until mixture is moist, rather than liquid – about 5 minutes. Season, and keep warm.

Meanwhile, make two deep slashes on each side of the mullet, brush with oil and season. Grill the mullet under a pre-heated grill, for about 4 minutes on each side until just cooked through. Serve with the chicory, scattered with the orange zest and a little chopped parsley.

Christian Fuentes' Honey-glazed Chicory

Christian Fuentes is French, but for the past eleven years he's made his home in London, working as a freelance chef. He remembers the first time he came across raw chicory in a salad. He was very surprised at what seemed to him a strange idea – as a boy he'd only ever eaten chicory cooked. Once he'd overcome the culture shock, he decided it wasn't a bad notion . . . but even so he still prefers his chicory hot and this is his favourite way of cooking it.

Now that I've tasted it, I think it could well become one of my favourite ways with chicory, too. Caramelized in a honey, butter and lemon syrup, the chicory is wonderfully sweet, sharp and mildly bitter all in one. Christian recommended serving it with fish, chicken or rabbit.

SERVES 6

6 medium heads of chicory
3 tablespoons honey
Juice of 1 lemon
25 g (1 oz) butter
Salt and freshly ground black pepper

Trim the chicory. Pack into a deep-sided frying-pan in a single layer. Drizzle honey and lemon juice over, add a little salt and dot with butter. Pour over enough water to almost cover. Cover and bring up to the boil. Uncover and simmer gently, turning once or twice until the water has virtually all evaporated leaving just a thick syrup. Start turning the chicory in the syrup as they begin to brown, so that they are nicely coated in the caramelized syrup. Whip off the heat before they burn and serve.

Endive au Jambon
[Chicory with Ham]

As far as I'm concerned, this is the way to cook chicory. I was brought up on Endive au jambon, and can eat it until the cows come home. Choose the best cooked ham, simmer the sauce until thick, and bake the gratin until browned and bubbling, and you will have before you one of the true French classics.

Notice, too, the curious linguistic twist: what we call chicory in English, is 'endive' in French, while our endive is . . . yes, that's right, 'chicorée'.

SERVES 4 as a first course, 2 as a main course

4 heads of chicory	450 ml (15 fl oz) milk
Squeeze of lemon juice	25 g (1 oz) grated Gruyère cheese
4 slices cooked ham	50 g (2 oz) freshly grated Parmesan
2 teaspoons Dijon mustard	cheese
40 g (1½ oz) butter	Salt, freshly ground black pepper and
½ onion, finely chopped	ground nutmeg
2 tablespoons plain flour	5 tablespoons breadcrumbs

Trim the chicory and cook in boiling salted water, acidulated with the lemon juice, until just tender but still firm at the centre. Drain really well squeezing out water. Spread the mustard over the ham, and roll each head of chicory in a slice of ham, with the mustard inside. Arrange closely together in buttered ovenproof dish.

Pre-heat the oven to gas mark 6, 400°F (200°C).

Melt 25 g (1 oz) of the butter in a saucepan and add the onion. Cook gently until tender, without browning. Sprinkle over the flour and stir to mix evenly. Cook for 1 minute, stirring. Gradually stir in the milk to give a smooth white sauce. Bring to the boil, and simmer for 10 minutes or so, stirring frequently, until thick and creamy. Stir in the Gruyère and half the Parmesan, salt, pepper and nutmeg to taste (season fairly generously). Pour over the chicory.

Mix the remaining Parmesan with the breadcrumbs, and sprinkle evenly over the top. Dot with the remaining butter. Bake until nicely browned and sizzling. Serve immediately.

Fried Radicchio

Though we tend to think of it as just another decorative leaf for salads, radicchio, like chicory, can be cooked very successfully. The drawback is that its dark cherry-pink colour fades to brown, but the taste makes up for that.

SERVES 4–6

2 heads of radicchio
2 tablespoons olive oil
50 g (2 oz) pancetta
  or streaky bacon, diced
1 clove garlic, peeled and finely
  chopped
Salt and freshly ground black pepper

Separate out the leaves of the radicchio and wash well. Drain as thoroughly as you can, then cut roughly into strips about 2.5 cm (1 inch) wide. Wrap in a clean tea towel until ready to cook.

Heat the oil in a frying-pan large enough to squash all the radicchio into. Fry the pancetta or bacon in the oil for a few seconds until it is opaque, then add the garlic and continue cooking until garlic and bacon begin to colour. Quickly add all the radicchio, salt and pepper, then slam on a lid (or a large plate) and turn down the heat slightly. Cook for about 10 minutes, stirring occasionally, until the radicchio has wilted. Taste and adjust seasonings and serve immediately.

Watercress

T he Watercress Line used to run from Alresford in Hampshire up to London. In its heyday the steam trains, laden with a cargo of leafy watercress packed in wicker baskets, sped up the line once a day when the season was at its height in springtime. Alresford is still one of the main watercress centres in the country and modern cultivation means that the season lasts the year round. Refrigerated lorries have replaced the steam trains, but the Watercress Line is not entirely defunct. Local enthusiasts band together throughout the summer to take the old trains along a few miles of track, serving a watercress lunch to customers as the scenery trundles past. The watercress arrives straight from the local beds, as fresh as a daisy, just the way it ought to be.

The peppery vigour of watercress injects instant liveliness into a green salad, but it's not so strong that it is unpleasant on its own. I like it too with chicory, orange and walnuts (see p. 193), a winter salad to relieve the stodgy tedium of cold weather food. As a garnish it should count as more than just a verdant frolic on the side of the plate. Traditionally tucked in around roast gamebirds, it plays an important role as a contrast to the gaminess of the fowl and the richness of other accompaniments. But as far as I'm concerned the best of all places for raw watercress is in a sandwich. Good brown bread, plenty of salted butter and a huge wodge of watercress. Bliss.

Landcress and wintercress are very like watercress, though with a stronger pepperiness. They both grow easily in gardens. Indian cress is another name for nasturtiums. Like the other cresses, they are peppery in taste. If you have tumbling nasturtiums in your flowerbeds or windowboxes, nip off a few leaves or flowers to embellish the next salad you make.

Chicken with Watercress Sauce

This is an elegant cream- and green-coloured dish, with a fresh gently peppery taste. I sometimes use the same method with fish, adjusting the timing to cook fillets or steaks as appropriate.

SERVES 4

1 bunch of watercress
25 g (1 oz) butter
1 tablespoon oil
4 chicken breasts, boned and skinned
1 shallot, finely chopped

Wine glass of dry white wine
150 ml (5 fl oz) double cream
Salt, freshly ground black pepper and
  nutmeg

Preparing Watercress

Whenever I can I buy watercress in tight bunches rather than sealed plastic bags. I like the look of it – far more aesthetically pleasing – but that's not the only reason. It's easy to tell at a glance the state of the watercress. There's no hiding yellowing leaves or smelly slimy stalks. Back in the kitchen the preparation is far quicker. To separate leaves from stalks is a simple matter of slicing down in a single stroke, close to the leaves for soups and sauces, a couple of inches down for longer sprigs. All they need then is a good rinse, thorough draining and to be dried gently with kitchen paper or a clean tea towel.

When you want to keep watercress for a couple of days, bunches are better, too. Plunge them into a bowl of water, leaves downwards, stems up in the air, and place in the fridge. Watercress stays perky and bright for far longer in this odd bottoms-up position.

Cooked watercress loses some of its peppery impact, but gives a good flavour to soups, sauces or stuffings. This is where the stems come into their own, adding substance as well as flavour. The leaves are best added right at the end of cooking time wherever feasible so that they retain as much as possible of their greenness and zip.

Strip the leaves off the watercress stalks discarding any damaged leaves (save stalks for soup). Set aside a dozen or so leaves for decoration, and chop the remainder fairly finely.

Melt the butter with the oil in a frying-pan just large enough to take the chicken breasts. When it is foaming, lay the chicken in the pan, brown lightly, then cover and cook over a moderate heat for 15–20 minutes, until it is just cooked through. Remove chicken and keep to one side.

Now add the chopped shallot to the pan and cook gently for 2–3 minutes until tender, without browning. Pour in the wine and let it bubble, scraping up the residues in the pan, until it is reduced to a scant tablespoonful or two. Draw off the heat, let the bubbles subside and then stir in the cream and the chopped watercress. Simmer for 5 minutes until reduced by about half. Season with salt, pepper, and a little nutmeg, then return the chicken to the pan and let it simmer for about 3 minutes so that it is thoroughly re-heated. Serve, scattered with reserved watercress leaves.

Watercress Soup

In France watercress soup is sometimes called 'potage santé' – health soup – which suggests that it is dull and worthy. Nothing could be further from the truth. This is a soup which is as good served cold as hot.

SERVES 4

1 bunch of watercress	1 clove garlic, peeled and chopped
50 g (2 oz) butter	450 g (1 lb) potatoes, peeled and diced
1 onion	600 ml (1 pint) water from cooking
1 bay leaf	vegetables *or* light stock
2 sprigs of thyme	Salt and freshly ground black pepper
2 sprigs of parsley	600 ml (1 pint) milk

Pick over and wash the watercress and discard any damaged leaves. Cut off the leaves, chop roughly and reserve. Chop the stalks. Melt the butter in a large saucepan, and add the onion, garlic, watercress stalks and herbs, tied in a bundle with string. Stir to coat nicely in butter, then cover and sweat over a low heat for 10 minutes. Now add the potatoes, water or stock, salt and pepper. Bring to the boil, and simmer for 20 minutes or so until the potato is tender. Remove the herbs.

Stir in half the milk and then the reserved watercress leaves. Process in batches until smooth. If you don't have a food processor, sieve the potato mixture, minus the leaves and milk. Mix in the milk, chop the watercress leaves finely and then add them too. Either way, return the mixture to the pan just before serving, adding the rest of the milk. Taste and adjust seasoning, then re-heat without boiling or serve chilled.

Watercress Sandwiches with Chilli Lemon Butter

Watercress sandwiches are one of the great delights of the world, in the same vein as and every bit as good as cucumber sandwiches. We used to have them for supper when I was a child. My father thought they should be made with white bread, but I preferred them with brown and still do. Brown or white, they have to be made with butter, not margarine, and you should pack a really generous quantity of watercress between the slices. No point in being niggardly.

Even better than plain butter is this flavoured butter. Quite how far the 50 g (2 oz) of flavoured butter will go depends on the size of the slices of bread, but there should be ample for at least three sandwiches and probably four.

Makes 3–4 sandwiches
1 bunch watercress
6–8 thin slices wholemeal
    or granary bread

For the butter
50 g (2 oz) lightly salted butter, softened
½ fresh green chilli, de-seeded and very
    finely chopped
Finely grated zest of ½ lemon
1 tablespoon lemon juice

To make the butter, process all the butter ingredients together. If you don't have or don't feel like using the processor, make sure that the chilli is very finely chopped indeed, then mash all ingredients together well with a fork. If you don't want to use the butter immediately, store, covered, in the fridge until needed. Bring back to room temperature before using.

Pick over and wash the watercress and remove any damaged leaves. Butter the bread fairly generously. Heap the watercress up really thickly on 3 or 4 slices and then clamp the upper slices down firmly, pressing into place. Cut in half and eat . . .

Radishes

If you thought radishes were just those little pink or pink and white things that are so nice to nibble at the beginning of a meal, then you've been missing out. Those are just two of a massive number of radish varieties. The almost spherical pink ones are probably Scarlet Globe or Pink Beauty, the longer pink and white ones will be French Breakfast, the commonest examples of summer radishes. There are two other categories of radish – winter and oriental. What's more every bit of the plant is edible, and that includes leaves and pods as well as roots.

The medieval town of Shrewsbury is home to the most astonishing radish collection I've ever seen. The curator is Adrian Jones, the location his allotment on the outskirts of town. The allotment is not solely dedicated to radishes – he grows all sorts of vegetables – but there are an awful lot of them. At last count, Adrian totted up some 20 different varieties dotted about in rows and clumps, a total made up of nine types of summer radish, three of winter radish, five oriental and three grown specifically for their leaves or pods.

Summer radishes are the easiest to grow and rewardingly speedy, reaching maturity within three to four weeks. Adrian Jones often leaves a few in the ground to run to flower and eventually to seed. The pods are almost as good as the radishes themselves, with a gentle peppery bite – excellent in salads or stir-fried.

Bisai is a curious radish. The roots are so spindly that they are not worth bothering with. But Bisai seeds are the best seeds for sprouting (though any radish seed will do), like alfalfa or mung beans. Planted out, they also produce a particularly fine crop of green leaves. Picked very young and small these are good in salads, and when fully grown they can be cooked and eaten like spinach.

The colossal winter and oriental radishes need a bit more love and attention. Though winter radishes can be eaten raw, I don't much care for the taste and prefer them cooked in much the same way as turnips (particularly good glazed with butter and sugar). The orientals are quite another matter. The long white mooli or daikon is frequently sold in shops and supermarkets, but visually it is about the least interesting of the orientals. Man Tang Hong and Rose Heart look even duller as they are pulled out of the earth, but slice them open and the interior is stunning – bright pink rosettes against white with a narrow band of bright green around the edge. They all taste deliciously sweet and nutty raw, and are very good cooked, too.

Preparing Summer Radishes

Buy radishes in bunches if possible, with lively green leaves. Trim off the long roots and the leaves (which can be saved to cook like spinach) leaving just a small tuft of green stems. Wash radishes thoroughly, then scrape away any clinging grit or scaly skin around the base of the stems. To keep them fresh and crisp, leave in a bowl of iced water until needed, then drain and serve with a pat of unsalted butter and coarse sea salt.

Sprouting Radishes

Sprouted radish seeds have a peppery taste that is very appealing in salads or sandwiches. You can sprout any summer radish seeds, though Bisai are particularly recommended. Wash the seeds well, and soak overnight. Rinse again. Place in jam jars, in a layer no more than 2.5 cm (1 inch) thick so that there is plenty of room for them to grow. Cover the top of the jar with muslin and secure with a rubber band. Lay the jar on its side in a roasting tin or shallow tray, with the bottom slightly raised so that excess water can drain away. Leave in a dark warm place, such as the airing cupboard. Rinse the seeds twice a day, so that they don't turn mouldy. After two or three days the sprouts should be 1 cm (½ inch) or so long. Bring the jar out into the light and give them 24 hours more, still rinsing, to turn them green. Rinse once more and eat within twenty four hours.

Raw Vegetable Pickles

These delicious Japanese pickles are best made 24–48 hours in advance. The red of the pepper and radishes (if you use red-skinned ones, that is) is gradually released to colour the turnip an enchanting shade of pink. They will keep for up to a week in the fridge.

20 pink summer radishes, sliced
    or 225-g (8-oz) piece of oriental
    radish (such as mooli, daikon or
    white radish), peeled and cut into
    matchsticks
2 large carrots, peeled and cut into
    matchsticks
2 turnips, peeled, halved and
    thinly sliced

1 cucumber, cut into matchsticks
1 red pepper, cut into thin strips
1 tablespoon salt
2 tablespoons sesame seeds
175 ml (6 fl oz) rice vinegar *or* white
    wine vinegar

Mix all the vegetables in a large bowl. Sprinkle with salt, and mix thoroughly with your hands to make sure that all the vegetables are evenly coated. Set aside for 15 minutes.

In a small heavy frying-pan, dry-fry the sesame seeds over a high heat, shaking the pan gently, until they begin to jump and give off a delicious nutty smell. Tip into a bowl and leave to cool.

Go back to the vegetables. Knead with your hands for a minute or two, then tip into a colander. Squeeze out as much liquid as you can, and transfer to a clean bowl. Add the vinegar and sesame seeds and mix well. Cover and leave in the fridge for at least 30 minutes, and up to 3 days, stirring occasionally. Covered, they will keep for up to a week in the fridge.

Oriental Radish with Miso Sauce

This is a popular Japanese way of serving oriental radish, steamed to tenderness and topped with a dollop of thick miso sauce. There are many different kinds of miso, a paste made from fermented soya beans and grains, varying in flavour from sweet and dense to dark and marmitey. Good healthfood shops and, naturally, Japanese food shops should stock the full range. Mirin is a sweet cooking wine, also available from Japanese food shops.

SERVES 4–6 as a first course
1 mooli (white radish), peeled

For the sauce
175 g (6 oz) sweet white miso
3 tablespoons sake *or* dry sherry
2 tablespoons mirin *or* sweet sherry
1 level tablespoon sugar
1 egg yolk
Finely grated zest of 1 lemon

Slice the radish into discs about 2 cm (¾ inch) thick. Steam (or boil in a light stock) for 30–40 minutes until the radish is slightly translucent.

When the radish is almost cooked, make the sauce. Put the miso into a bowl and set over a pan of gently simmering water. Stir in the sake (or dry sherry) and mirin (or sweet sherry), then the sugar and egg yolk. Stir for a couple of minutes, until creamy and thick. If it gets too thick too quickly, add a splash of water. Finally stir in the lemon zest.

Arrange the radish slices on plates, and top with a generous dollop of the warm sauce. Serve immediately.

Braised Oriental Radish with Black Beans

Braised gently with salted black beans, chillies and other oriental flavourings, oriental radish takes on a distinctly new character. Hot and spicy, this will make you appreciate the radish in a totally new way.

SERVES 4

450 g (1 lb) mooli (white radish), peeled
2 tablespoons sunflower *or* vegetable oil
4 spring onions, chopped
1-cm (½-inch) piece fresh ginger, peeled and finely chopped
2 cloves garlic, peeled and finely chopped
1 green chilli, de-seeded and finely chopped
1 tablespoon Chinese salted black beans, rinsed
2 tablespoons dark soy sauce
1 tablespoon rice vinegar
   or white wine vinegar
2 teaspoons sugar
½ star anise
300 ml (10 fl oz) chicken
   or vegetable stock

Slice the radish into 5-mm (¼-inch) thick discs, then quarter the discs.

Heat the oil in a wok or deep frying-pan until it smokes. Quickly add the spring onion, ginger, garlic and chilli and stir-fry for a few seconds. Add the radish and black beans and stir-fry for about 1 minute. Add all the remaining ingredients, bring to the boil, stirring, then cover and simmer for 20–30 minutes until the radish is almost tender. Uncover and boil for a few minutes until the sauce is reduced. Serve.

GREENS

Brussels Sprouts • Cabbage • Spinach
Broccoli • Cauliflower • Chard

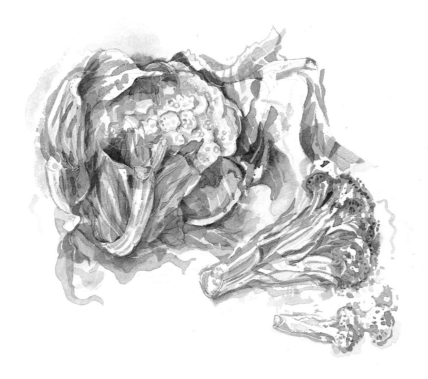

Brussels Sprouts

F rench chef Christian Germain fell for his English wife, Lyndsey, and Brussels sprouts while he was working in this country. He took them both back to France with him when he returned to set up his own hotel and restaurant in the small, walled town of Montreuil near Boulogne – Lyndsey as co-proprietor, sprouts firmly relegated to the garden. Picked small, and tightly furled on crisp autumn and winter mornings, the Brussels sprouts reach the diners in a state of absolute perfection. They have been a *succès fou*. The French clients adore them and the Château de Montreuil is renowned locally for the novel deliciousness of chef Germain's vegetables.

Brussels sprouts are a peculiarly British phenomenon. Miniature cabbages clinging in knobbly rows up a tough stalk, they are the strangest-looking brassicas of all as they grow. When they are small, fresh, and not overcooked Brussels sprouts can be very good. When they are on the large side, days away from the plant, and overcooked they are foul.

Fried Brussels Sprouts

. . . or Brussels sprouts in disguise. They are certainly not recognizable cooked like this, not visually and possibly not tastewise, either. If you have a deep-rooted passion for sprouts then this may be no great recommendation. Personally, I find them much more interesting cooked this way than practically any other, with the exception of the two recipes that follow. Shredding the sprouts is a mite boring, but it won't take that long, and the speediness with which they cook makes up amply for lost time.

SERVES 4
450 g (1 lb) Brussels sprouts
2 tablespoons olive oil
2 cloves garlic, peeled and
    finely chopped
Salt and freshly ground black pepper
1 tablespoon chopped fresh parsley

Shred the Brussels sprouts finely. Heat the oil in a wide frying-pan and add the garlic and sprouts. Sauté over a moderate heat until the sprouts are lightly patched with brown. Season with salt and pepper. Sprinkle with parsley and serve.

Preparing Brussels Sprouts

Never buy Brussels sprouts that are loose-leaved or floppy and yellowing. Not only are they well past their best, but they are also likely to harbour small insects which makes cleaning them a chore. With tiny, tight spheres all you need do is trim off the outer leaves and a thin slice of the base. Don't bother cutting crosses in the base – quite unnecessary and it doubles preparation time. Steam or cook in a small amount of water until they are just tender but slightly firm in the centre, so that they keep their nutty flavour without becoming rank-tasting. If the worst comes to the worst and they are overcooked the best thing to do is to purée them with butter, a little cream or milk, salt, freshly ground black pepper and plenty of nutmeg.

To make Brussels sprouts even nicer, cook them in water until almost done, drain well and fry in butter until lightly patched with brown. At Christmas time add cooked chestnuts to the pan too. Look out for the pretty red Brussels sprouts, which have a fine, nutty sweetness.

Stoved Brussels Sprouts and Carrots

Overcooking any member of the brassicas is a sin, but one that is turned into a virtue if you just keep right on cooking. That's the theory here, and it works, too. Braised together for 45 minutes or so, Brussels sprouts and carrots simmer gently down to a remarkably happy union of flavour. Don't be tempted to stir too energetically, as sprouts are tender things and will end up fuzzier than they should.

SERVES 6

50 g (2 oz) butter
750 g (1½ lb) Brussels sprouts, trimmed
450 g (1 lb) carrots, peeled and cut into
    1-cm (½-inch) slices

1 onion, chopped
½ teaspoon dried rosemary
½ teaspoon dried thyme
Salt and freshly ground black pepper

In a wide, heavy frying-pan, melt the butter. Add the Brussels sprouts, carrots, onion, herbs, salt and pepper. Almost, but not quite, cover the vegetables with water. Bring to a gentle simmer, then cover (use a large plate if you don't have a big enough saucepan lid). Simmer very gently, stirring occasionally, for 30 minutes.

Remove the lid and raise the heat slightly. Let it simmer, stirring frequently, until most of the water has evaporated leaving just a thin layer on the base of the pan. Taste and check seasoning and serve, or leave to cool and re-heat when needed. You may need to add a couple of tablespoons of water to prevent sticking when re-heating.

Brussels Sprouts with Bacon, Almonds and Cream

As far as I'm concerned, this is a recipe with CHRISTMAS LUNCH *written large across it. It's about as decadent as you can get with a pound and a half of Brussels sprouts and just the thing to dish up with the roast turkey. Mind you, it tastes so good that it would be a shame to eat it only once a year.*

SERVES 6

750 g (1½ lb) small Brussels sprouts
15 g (½ oz) butter
1 tablespoon oil
1 × 100-g (4-oz) piece of smoked back
    bacon *or* thick-cut bacon, diced
15 g (½ oz) flaked almonds
175 ml (6 fl oz) double cream
Finely grated zest of ½ lemon
Salt and freshly ground black pepper
Dash of lemon juice

Trim the sprouts, and drop into a saucepan of boiling salted water. Simmer until almost but not quite cooked, then drain thoroughly and pat dry with kitchen paper.

Heat the butter and oil in a wide frying-pan. Add the bacon and almonds and sauté until lightly browned. Add the sprouts and cook for 2–3 more minutes, stirring. Draw off the heat, cool for a few seconds, then add the double cream and lemon zest. Return to the heat and let the cream bubble, stirring frequently, for about 4 minutes until reduced to a rich sauce. Off the heat, season with salt, pepper and a dash of lemon juice. Serve immediately.

Cabbage

We walked into a pub in search of lunch and walked straight out again. It was the smell of stale fat and overcooked cabbage that we couldn't stomach, hungry as we were. These are two of the nastiest and most pervasive of kitchen smells, ones that linger as a sure sign that all is not well on the food front.

Cabbage should be cooked in one of two ways: very briefly in the minimum of water, or very lengthily in the minimum of water, if any at all. Anything in between is a mistake best avoided. I found a scientific explanation for this in food-scientist Harold McGee's book *On food and cooking*; as cabbage is cooked, compounds including ammonia and hydrogen sulphide – the rotten egg smell – are produced. Between the fifth and seventh minute of cooking the amount of hydrogen sulphide doubles in output. So, either get your cabbage cooked in less than 5 minutes, or keep going for long enough for all the chemical changes to take place and the less favourable flavours and smells to be cooked off.

When choosing cabbage of whatever type, look for fresh leaves with few blemishes (ignore any with yellowing leaves), and a solid, firm centre. The cabbage should feel heavy for its size. If it is in fine fettle to start with it will keep for up to a week in the vegetable drawer of the fridge, or in a cool dark place.

Slow-cooked Cabbage with Lemon

Stewed very slowly for an hour or more in its own juices with a generous knob of butter, dull white cabbage takes on a whole new persona. It softens down to a nutty, mellow flavour. When I was in Ireland, I nervously tried this one out on a hungry truck-driver in Mother Hubbard's diner. 'Scrumptious,' he said as he polished off his helping, and that about sums it up.

Serves 4–6

1 kg (2 lb) white cabbage	2 teaspoons sugar
1 lemon	Salt and freshly ground black pepper
75 g (3 oz) lightly salted butter	

Slice the cabbage into strips about 1 cm (½ inch) wide, discarding the tough core. Pare the zest from the lemon in wide strips, and squeeze out the juice. Melt the butter in a saucepan large enough to take all the cabbage. Add cabbage, lemon zest, sugar, salt and pepper. Turn to mix, then cover tightly and cook over a low heat for 1 hour, stirring occasionally, until

Preparing Cabbage

The usual way to prepare white, green and red cabbage is to remove outer leaves if necessary, then cut into quarters and remove the tough stalk before shredding or slicing, though for stuffing, you will want to keep the leaves whole. To cook, wash the shredded or sliced leaves briefly and put into a pan with a knob of butter, salt and just enough water to prevent burning. Clamp on the lid and cook over a high heat for a few minutes, turning occasionally, until softened. Only when blanching leaves for stuffing should you drop them, for as short a time as you can get away with, into a large saucepan of boiling water.

The classic way to cook red cabbage is long and slow, with sweet and sour additions – a cooking apple, raisins, sugar or honey, vinegar or red wine, and orange juice. It's a marvellous dish, but I've not given a recipe for it as there are so many around that you will have no difficulty finding one if you don't already have your own version. Instead, I've suggested stir-frying which is much quicker.

Savoy cabbage is the beauty of this group, with its dark green crinkled leaves and pale ribs. In taste too I think it the best, with less of the rankness usually associated with cabbages. For this reason it can take brief boiling in large amounts of water as long as it is well drained, but it is nicer cooked with minimal water. I love it shredded and added to soups for the last few minutes of simmering, and it is the best choice for stuffing.

the cabbage is meltingly tender and all the liquid it has exuded has been reabsorbed or evaporated. If it still seems a little watery after an hour, remove the lid and let it burble quietly for another 5–10 minutes. Now add the lemon juice, cover and cook for a few minutes longer. Taste, adjust seasonings and serve.

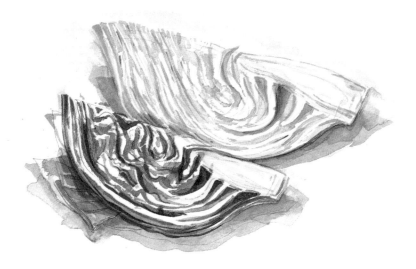

Colcannon

On the road from Dublin to the west coast of Ireland, not far from Mullingar in County Westmeath, is Mother Hubbard's Diner, a celebrated truckers' stop, where the food is good and wholesome, the surroundings are spruce and clean and the atmosphere cheerful and welcoming. At Mother Hubbard's they grow their own cabbages in the vegetable patch alongside the diner, together with herbs and rhubarb for making pies. Trish Doyle, who runs the diner, cooked Colcannon for me, the traditional Irish dish of mashed potato and cabbage. It used to be served at Hallowe'en, with lucky charms buried deep inside the steaming, pale green mound. Whoever found the ring would be married within the year, while the coin promised a great fortune.

SERVES 6

450 g (1 lb) trimmed green cabbage
  or curly kale
300 ml (10 fl oz) full cream milk
  or better still, single cream
50 g (2 oz) butter

2 large onions *or* 2 large leeks
  or 8 spring onions, chopped
450 g (1 lb) floury potatoes
Salt and freshly ground black pepper

Boil the cabbage in salted water for 20–30 minutes until very tender. Squeeze dry, then chop roughly. Put the milk, or cream, and butter into a saucepan with the onions, leeks or spring onions and simmer for 20 minutes.

Boil the potatoes in their skins. Drain thoroughly, peel and mash. Process or liquidize the milk/cream and onions/leeks/spring onion mixture with the cabbage until fairly smooth. Beat into the mashed potato. Taste, season and re-heat gently if necessary.

Pasta with Savoy Cabbage and Shallots

The mixture of cabbage, caraway seeds and pasta may sound somewhat unpromising, but in practice it works brilliantly to produce an unusual but delicious pasta dish. No cheese with this one please.

SERVES 2

25 g (1 oz) butter
2 shallots, sliced
2 cloves garlic, peeled and sliced
1 teaspoon caraway seeds

6 leaves Savoy cabbage, shredded
Salt and freshly ground black pepper
Paprika
225 g (8 oz) tagliatelle

Melt the butter in a medium-sized saucepan. Add the shallots, garlic and caraway seeds. Cover and cook over a low heat for 5 minutes, stirring once or twice to prevent catching. Add the Savoy cabbage, salt, pepper and a shake of paprika. Cover again, and cook for a further 5 minutes, stirring occasionally, until the cabbage has wilted.

Bring a large pan of salted water to the boil. Drop in the tagliatelle, and bring back to the boil. Simmer until *al dente*. Drain and toss with cabbage and shallot mixture and all the buttery juices. Serve immediately.

Cabbage, Onion and Dolcelatte Tian

A tian is a French gratin dish with sloping sides so that you get the maximum possible expanse of crusty brown top. The word has also come to mean what is cooked in the dish.

SERVES 6

2 large onions, thinly sliced
1 clove garlic, peeled and chopped
2 tablespoons olive oil
1 small Savoy cabbage
3 eggs, beaten

150 ml (5 fl oz) milk
100 g (4 oz) dolcelatte cheese, crumbled
2 tablespoons chopped fresh parsley
Salt and freshly ground black pepper

Fry the onions and garlic gently in the oil until tender, without browning. Whilst they are cooking, shred the cabbage finely, discarding damaged outer leaves and the tough inner core. Bring a large saucepan of water to the boil, and drop in the cabbage. Bring back to the boil and simmer for 2 minutes. Drain and run under the cold tap. Drain again, press to expel excess moisture, then pat dry on kitchen paper.

Pre-heat the oven to gas mark 3, 325°F (160°C). Mix the cabbage with the onion and garlic. Beat the eggs lightly into the milk and pour into the vegetables, adding the dolcelatte, parsley and salt and pepper. Mix well. Spoon into an oiled 30-cm (12-inch) gratin dish, or other ovenproof dish to give a layer about 2.5 cm (1 inch) thick.

Bake for 40–50 minutes until set and browned on top. Eat hot or warm.

Stir-fried Sweet and Sour Red Cabbage

Stir-frying is one of the best methods to cook so many vegetables, and I find myself stir-frying all manner of things, often with not a hint of a Chinese flavour.

Don't be tempted to skip the salting of the cabbage. It draws out some of the water content, which means that it will cook more quickly, without stewing in its own juices.

SERVES 4–5

½ head of red cabbage
1 teaspoon salt
1½ tablespoons sunflower oil
2 tablespoons sherry vinegar
   or red wine vinegar

1 tablespoon water
1 tablespoon caster sugar
15 g (½ oz) pine kernels
25 g (1 oz) raisins
Freshly ground black pepper

Cut the tough central stalk out of the cabbage, then shred thinly. Spread out in a colander, and sprinkle with the salt. Turn, then leave to drain for 30 minutes. Rinse under the cold tap and pat dry with kitchen paper. Mix the vinegar with the water and sugar.

Heat the oil in a wok, or a large frying-pan until very hot. Keep the heat high throughout. Add the cabbage, and stir and toss for 3 minutes. Add the pine kernels and continue to stir-fry for 2 minutes. Stir the vinegar mixture, and pour into the cabbage. Add the raisins and plenty of pepper. Stir-fry for 1–2 minutes longer until the liquid has evaporated, and serve.

Spinach

Generations of children have been forced to eat spinach. 'It's good for you . . . full of iron.' Whether they liked it or not was neither here nor there. I was one of the lucky ones. I adored spinach and I doubt that my mother would have made me eat it if I hadn't. Those that did suffer may be interested to know that their parents were wrong. Not entirely, to be fair. Spinach *is* good for you and it does contain a lot of iron, but it is the vitamins A and C that are the healthy bit and you could have got them from carrots and strawberries. The iron is almost totally useless; it is 'bound' by the oxalic acid in spinach, which means that your body absorbs precious little of it – no more than 5 per cent. So much for adult wisdom. So much for Popeye.

Oxalic acid has a lot to answer for, as it may well be what puts many people off spinach in the first place, and rhubarb too. This is the substance that 'furs' up your mouth and teeth, setting them on edge. The level varies from one batch of spinach to another. I don't find it a problem, unless I over-indulge (the effect builds up as you eat), but then it serves me right for being greedy.

I'm an out-and-out spinach fan. I love it fresh – raw or cooked. The one thing I'm not keen on is frozen chopped spinach which is horribly mushy and slimy. Though I keep a bag of frozen leaf spinach in the freezer for emergencies, it really is much better when fresh, and it barely takes any more time to prepare and cook.

Medea Walker's Burani-ey-Esfinaj
[Spinach with Yoghurt]

Persian cooking is one of the great cuisines of the Middle East and spinach features heavily. The three recipes which follow were cooked for me by Medea Walker, a vivacious, glamorous Iranian whose family originates from a semi-desert area of Iran, where herds of animals are kept for meat, but fresh vegetables are a rare luxury. Spinach, in particular, is considered a great delicacy. The style of cooking of the region is less sophisticated than you might find in the cities and uses intriguingly different flavours and seasonings. This spinach and yoghurt dish is one of a whole feast of foods which might be prepared the day before a celebration. (Medea also makes a beetroot burani in exactly the same way.) Try to find sumac, the pleasingly sour-tasting Persian spice, but if you can't, use a little sweet paprika instead, for colour.

Preparing Spinach

Decent fresh spinach, the only sort worth forking out for, has a bouncy, squeaky look about it. There are bound to be a few damaged leaves to discard, but make sure that there are no more than the odd one or two. If you must keep it for more than a day, store it in a plastic bag in the fridge, but for no more than a couple of days. To prepare, snip off the thick stalks, then rinse thoroughly in several changes of water – spinach can be extremely gritty – discarding damaged leaves as you do so.

Shake the spinach to get rid of excess water but don't dry. Pack it tightly into a large saucepan and cover. You don't need to add any extra water. Cook over a low heat for a few minutes to get the juices running. Then raise the heat and give the spinach a quick stir. Cover again and cook for another 2–5 minutes, stirring once, until all the spinach has wilted down. Drain it thoroughly, pressing to get rid of excess water. 1 kg (2 lb) of spinach collapses down to 450 g (1 lb) in the pan, about enough for four of you. This is roughly equivalent to 750 g (1½ lb) unthawed frozen spinach.

When you are going to chop cooked spinach, or serve it in a sauce or some more complicated dish, it is doubly important to squeeze out as much water as is humanly possible. I usually do this by clamping the spinach between two identical upside down dinner plates and squeezing them firmly together. The juice will run out on all sides, so do it over a sink and with your sleeves rolled up well past your elbows.

Fresh, uncooked spinach responds well to stir-frying. The intense heat sizzles up the copious juices as they hit the sides of the wok. Cut the spinach into wide strips before you throw it into the oil. For salads, choose small-leaved spinach which is crisp and delicate, rather than the larger leaves which may be too strongly flavoured and tough.

SERVES 6

1 onion, chopped
2 tablespoons sunflower oil
225 g (8 oz) cooked spinach, roughly chopped

600 ml (1 pint) Greek-style yoghurt
1 clove garlic, peeled and crushed
Salt and freshly ground black pepper

To garnish
Powdered sumac *or* sweet paprika
Dried mint

Sauté the onion in the oil until browned. Cool slightly. Mix with the spinach, yoghurt, garlic, salt and pepper. Spoon into a serving bowl and chill until nearly ready to serve. Decorate the surface with a scattering of sumac or sweet paprika, and dried mint.

Kuku-ey-Esfinaj
[Baked Spinach Omelette]

When Medea Walker made me her Spinach burani (see p. 213), she also showed me two other spinach dishes. A kuku is an Iranian baked omelette packed full of vegetables. She flavours the kuku either with garlic, or with a mixture of herbs and spice, but never both. Either way, it makes a superb dish for a party, served with a bowl of yoghurt, or maybe a beetroot burani, and it is an ideal candidate for picnics and packed lunches.

SERVES 6–8

1 onion, chopped
2 tablespoons oil
25 g (1 oz) butter
450 g (1 lb) cooked spinach, squeezed
   dry and coarsely chopped
6 eggs

2 cloves garlic, peeled and crushed
   or ¼ teaspoon cinnamon and
   2 teaspoons dried dill and
   2 tablespoons chopped fresh coriander
Salt and freshly ground black pepper

Pre-heat the oven to gas mark 3, 325°F (160°C).

Fry the onion in the oil until browned. Add the butter and when melted, add the spinach, garlic or cinnamon, dill and coriander. Stir for 2–3 minutes until all the butter is absorbed, and everything is evenly mixed. Tip into a bowl and cool slightly, then beat in the eggs one at a time. Spoon into a *thoroughly* greased baking tin or dish, to give a layer about 2.5 cm (1 inch) thick. Cover with foil and bake for about 35–40 minutes until set, removing the foil after the first 20 minutes. Serve cool, cut into squares.

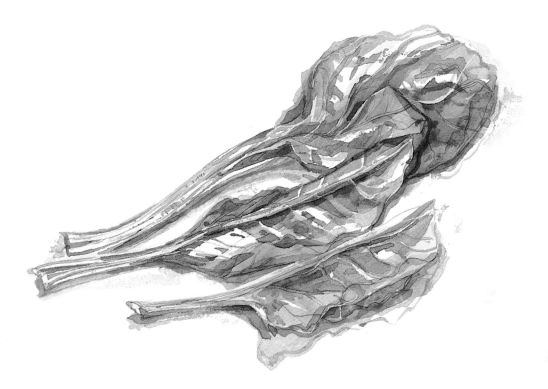

Esfinaj-en-Aloo
[Spinach with Apricots or Prunes]

This is probably the most bizarre-sounding recipe of the whole book – something I would never have dreamt up in my wildest dream. Still, Iranian cooking is justifiably famous, so when Medea Walker offered me a bowl of Esfinaj-en-aloo, I tried it without hesitation.

It is extraordinary, and strange and delicious. The spinach is cooked so long that it melts down, blending with the sweet sourness of the fruit. It won't be everyone's cup of tea, but I urge you to try it at least once.

If you are lucky, you may find sour pomegranate sauce in Middle Eastern food stores. It's a wonderful tart fruity sauce, good in meat stews as well as in this recipe. If you can't lay your hands on it, you'll have to make do with a mixture of black treacle and lemon juice. Rosewater is far easier to find, either expensively packaged in delicatessens, or more cheaply in Greek food shops, or more cheaply still at the chemist's where you should ask for triple strength rosewater.

SERVES 4

1 kg (2 lb) fresh spinach
or 450 g (1 lb) frozen leaf spinach
2 tablespoons oil
1 onion, chopped
25 g (1 oz) butter
2 cloves garlic, peeled, halved and crushed with a knife
350 g (12 oz) mushrooms, chopped

1½ tablespoons pomegranate sauce
or 1 tablespoon lemon juice
and 1 tablespoon black treacle
Pinch of ground saffron (*optional*)
Salt and freshly ground black pepper
225 g (8 oz) dried apricots *or* prunes
1 tablespoon rosewater (*optional*)

If using fresh spinach, wash and cook lightly. If using frozen leaf spinach, just let it thaw. Either way, drain thoroughly squeezing out water.

Heat the oil in a frying-pan and sauté the onion until browned. Add the butter and when melted, add the spinach, garlic and mushrooms. Cook over a fairly high heat, stirring constantly for about 4 minutes. Now stir in the pomegranate sauce, or the lemon juice and treacle, the saffron, salt and pepper. Finally, stir in the apricots or prunes and mix thoroughly. Transfer to a heavy casserole and add the rosewater, and enough water to cover generously. Cover with a lid and cook over the lowest possible heat (use a diffuser mat if you have one) for about 1¼–1½ hours, until very thick and rich. Taste and adjust seasoning, then leave to cool. Serve cold.

Spinach with Seville Orange and Breadcrumbs

The spicy sourness of Seville oranges adds a wonderful zest to spinach, but sadly their season is short. There is a year-round alternative, though it is not quite the same. When the marmalade-making season is over, substitute the juice of ½ lemon mixed with the juice of ½ ordinary orange for the Seville orange juice, and serve with wedges of orange.

SERVES 4

1 kg (2 lb) fresh spinach	Juice of 1 Seville orange
40 g (1½ oz) butter	1 teaspoon ground cinnamon
1 tablespoon sunflower oil	Salt and freshly ground black pepper
15 g (½ oz) fine dry breadcrumbs	4 wedges of Seville orange to serve

Wash the spinach thoroughly and discard any thick tough stems or damaged leaves. Shake off excess water, and pack the spinach into a large pan. Cover and cook over a gentle heat for 5 minutes. Stir, and cover again. Turn the heat up slightly, and cook for another 5−10 minutes, stirring occasionally until the spinach is just cooked. Drain well.

Heat 15 g (½ oz) of butter and the oil in a small frying-pan, and fry the breadcrumbs until golden brown. Drain on kitchen paper. Just before serving, re-heat the spinach with the remaining butter, Seville orange juice, cinnamon, salt and pepper, stirring as it heats up. Taste and adjust seasonings. At the same time, re-heat the breadcrumbs.

Tip the spinach into a serving dish, and scatter the crumbs over the top. Serve with orange wedges.

Cypriot Dried Broad Beans with Spinach

The woman who gave me this recipe used to run the curious ramshackle shop at the end of my road. It was a scruffy little place selling sweets, cigarettes and an odd collection of mainly Greek Cypriot provisions. The only time I ever saw her smile was when I bought a packet of dried skinned broad beans. She wanted to know how I was going to use them, and proffered this recipe in exchange. The shop has closed, the woman has disappeared, and I now have to go further afield to a far more impressive Greek food shop to buy the beans for this salad.

SERVES 6−8

175 g (6 oz) dried skinned broad beans, soaked overnight and drained	450 g (1 lb) spinach, washed and roughly chopped
1 onion, chopped	2−3 cloves garlic, peeled and crushed
8 tablespoons olive oil	2−3 tablespoons lemon juice
	Salt and freshly ground black pepper

Cook the broad beans in unsalted, boiling water until just tender (30–50 minutes). Drain. Meanwhile, fry the onion in 2 tablespoons of olive oil in a large saucepan until tender. Add the spinach, packing it in. Cover and cook over a gentle heat until the spinach begins to exude liquid. Stir, then raise the heat to moderate, uncover and continue cooking and stirring for a few minutes longer until the spinach has wilted. Draw off the heat, drain off excess liquid, and mix with the cooked beans, remaining oil, garlic, lemon juice, salt and pepper. Turn into a shallow dish and leave to cool. Taste and adjust seasonings, adding a little more oil or lemon as needed. Serve at room temperature.

Summer Vegetable Terrine

Spinach works well as a wrapping for terrines of all kinds, but is particularly appropriate for this light, fresh summer terrine of fennel, asparagus and courgettes set in a jellied tomato sauce. Allow plenty of time for making it – the layers have to be built up and left to set individually. Be patient. It's worth it in the end.

SERVES 8 as a first course

175 g (6 oz) thin asparagus	1 litre (1¾ pints) passata *or* liquidized
1 large fennel bulb	tinned tomatoes
175 g (6 oz) small courgettes	175 ml (6 fl oz) dry white wine
340 g (12 oz) fresh large-leafed spinach	12 large fresh basil leaves, roughly torn up
1 onion, chopped	1 teaspoon dried oregano
3 cloves garlic, peeled and chopped	Salt and freshly ground black pepper
1½ tablespoons olive oil	2 sachets powdered gelatine

Trim the asparagus. Slice off the base and stalks of fennel and cut into thin wedges. Halve or quarter the courgettes lengthwise. Steam or simmer all vegetables separately until tender. Drain, cool and cover until needed.

Fry the onion and garlic gently in the olive oil until tender. Add the passata or liquidized tomatoes, wine, oregano, salt and pepper and simmer for 10 minutes. Add the basil then liquidize and sieve. Adjust seasonings. Sprinkle the gelatine evenly over 6 tablespoons of hot water in a small saucepan and leave for 3 minutes. Warm gently, without boiling, stirring until the gelatine has dissolved. Draw off the heat and stir in 3 tablespoons of the warm tomato sauce. If any lumps form return to the heat for a few seconds. Mix well with the remaining sauce.

Trim the stalks from the spinach, and drop into a large saucepan of boiling water. Bring back to the boil, drain and spread out on kitchen paper to dry. Line a 1.75-litre (3-pint) long loaf tin with clingfilm and brush with oil. Line with spinach leaves, letting them flap over the top. Spoon in a quarter of the sauce, arrange the fennel on top. Chill, loosely covered until just set. Repeat layers using asparagus, then courgettes, chilling each time to let the sauce set, then cover with the remaining sauce. Flip over the trailing spinach leaves to cover, and chill until set. To serve, turn out, peel off clingfilm, and slice thickly with a sharp knife.

Broccoli

When my mother wrote her *Vegetable Book* in the late seventies, fresh plump green heads of broccoli calabrese (i.e. broccoli from Calabria where it was developed) were relative newcomers in shops and supermarkets. It was sold as calabrese to distinguish it from purple-sprouting broccoli which was far more widely known. Broccoli calabrese made a huge impact, soon ousting its older spindlier brother from a position of supremacy. For people of my generation and younger, broccoli invariably means the thick-stemmed newcomer, the name calabrese has been dropped, and purple-sprouting broccoli is now the more unusual of the two.

Smothered Broccoli with White Wine

Forget al dente for the moment — in this recipe the broccoli is cooked long and slow until meltingly tender, bringing out the full sweetness of the vegetable. It is so good that it should be savoured on its own as a first course, though it would make a good partner too, to a meaty main course.

SERVES 4–6 as a first course or side dish

750 g (1½ lb) broccoli
2 dried red chillies
5 tablespoons olive oil
6 cloves garlic, peeled
6 pieces of sun-dried tomato, cut into thin strips *or* 10 black olives, halved and pitted

Salt and freshly ground black pepper
250 ml (8 fl oz) dry white wine
40 g (1½ oz) fresh Parmesan cheese, sliced into paper-thin shavings

Cut off the tough, woody ends of the broccoli stems. Leave thinner stems up to 1-cm (½-inch) whole, cut thicker ones in half or quarters along their length. Cut each piece in half. Break chillies into pieces and shake out the seeds. Cover the base of a wide, deep, heavy frying-pan, or saucepan, with a thin layer of olive oil. Cover with a thick layer of the broccoli, scatter over half the garlic, the sun-dried tomato or olives, the chilli, salt and pepper, and half the remaining olive oil. Repeat the layers. Pour over the wine. Cover and cook over a very gentle heat for 40 minutes to 1 hour until the liquid has almost all evaporated, removing the lid towards the end of cooking if necessary. Spoon into a serving dish, and scatter with shavings of Parmesan. Serve immediately.

Preparing Broccoli

The appearance of the first bundles of purple-sprouting broccoli in late winter is an event I look forward to. As long as they are stiff and fresh – floppy old stems are not worth bothering with – they need little preparation. Trim off the woody base of the stems, remove any damaged leaves and give them a good rinse. Some people strip off all the leaves, but this seems a terrible waste. I find it easiest to steam purple-sprouting broccoli. The alternative is to cook it like asparagus: tie the shoots in bundles and stand them upright in enough boiling, salted water to come about half-way up the stems. Cover tightly and cook until the stems are tender. The stems will be boiled, but the delicate heads are steamed. If you have an asparagus steamer use that, otherwise wedge them upright with scrumpled silver foil. Serve with melted butter and a dash of orange or lemon juice, or with an orange-flavoured Hollandaise. They make a delicious salad too, turned carefully in vinaigrette.

It is a mistake to steam broccoli proper (by which I mean calabrese). It tastes fine, but it turns a grim murky green that is far from attractive. Instead, I either boil or microwave it so that it retains its bright colour. I've been shocked to hear that some people throw away large parts of the stalk. It's the best bit!

I have two stock ways of preparing broccoli. Both begin with trimming the base and paring off the outer skin on the lower part of the stem if it seems tough. Sometimes, I'll divide the thick stems and flowering heads lengthwise into long strips which I cook whole, lying down in water. As long as you don't overdo matters, the heads are firm enough to survive undamaged. Sometimes, I slice the stem about 1 cm (½ inch) thick, and separate the head into small florets. The stem pieces go into the water first, followed after 2–3 minutes by the florets. Four or five minutes later they will all be done nicely. Perfectly cooked broccoli is tender, but firm and sweet, never ever mushy or watery.

Broccoli with Chilli and Parmesan

This is a quick way to dress up cooked broccoli with a dash of fire. Spiked with chilli and garlic, melting slivers of Parmesan on top, it's a nifty way to transform broccoli into something special.

SERVES 4

750 g (1½ lb) broccoli
Salt
3 tablespoons olive oil
¼–½ teaspoon chilli flakes

2–3 cloves garlic, peeled and finely chopped
15 g (½ oz) Parmesan cheese, cut into paper-thin slivers

Separate the broccoli florets from the stalks. Slice the stalks about 1 cm (½ inch) thick. Drop the stalks into a pan of lightly salted boiling water. Simmer for 2 minutes, then add the florets and cook for a further 2–3 minutes until almost but not quite done. Drain, run under the cold tap to refresh then leave to drain completely and pat dry on kitchen paper.

Heat the oil in a wide frying-pan, and add the chilli and garlic. Cook over a low heat for about 1 minute, then add the broccoli. Raise the heat a little and stir and fry for 4–5 minutes until the broccoli is piping hot. Tip into a serving dish and scatter over the Parmesan. Serve at once.

Smoked Haddock Pasties

Lovely hot from the oven and almost as good cold, perhaps for a packed lunch or a picnic, these pasties are filled with a moist mixture of smoked haddock, broccoli and tomato.

MAKES 6 pasties

450 g (1 lb) undyed smoked haddock fillet
1 bay leaf
3 peppercorns
2 sprigs fresh parsley
Milk
350 g (12 oz) broccoli
2 tablespoons olive oil *or* sunflower oil

2 cloves garlic, peeled and chopped
350 g (12 oz) tomatoes, skinned, de-seeded and roughly chopped
½ teaspoon dried thyme
Salt and freshly ground black pepper
750 g (1½ lb) shortcrust pastry (see p. 20)
1 egg, beaten

Put the haddock, cut into two or three pieces if necessary, in a frying-pan with the bay leaf, peppercorns and parsley. Add enough milk and water in equal quantities just to cover the fish. Bring to a simmer then reduce the heat and poach until the haddock is tender. Drain, then skin and flake, removing any bones.

Slice the stems of the broccoli and separate the head into small florets. Cook in salted boiling water for 3–4 minutes until *al dente*. Drain thoroughly.

Heat the oil in a frying-pan, add the garlic, tomatoes and thyme and cook briskly for 5 minutes or so until the tomatoes have collapsed to make a very thick sauce, with no trace of wateriness. Stir in the haddock and broccoli and draw off the heat. Season with pepper and salt if needed (smoked haddock can be quite salty, so go carefully). Cool until tepid.

Divide the pastry into 6 and roll each piece out to give a circle of about 18 cm (7 inches) in diameter. Mound a sixth of the filling in the centre of each circle. Brush the edges with

OVERLEAF *Parcels of Cauliflower and Broccoli Cheese*

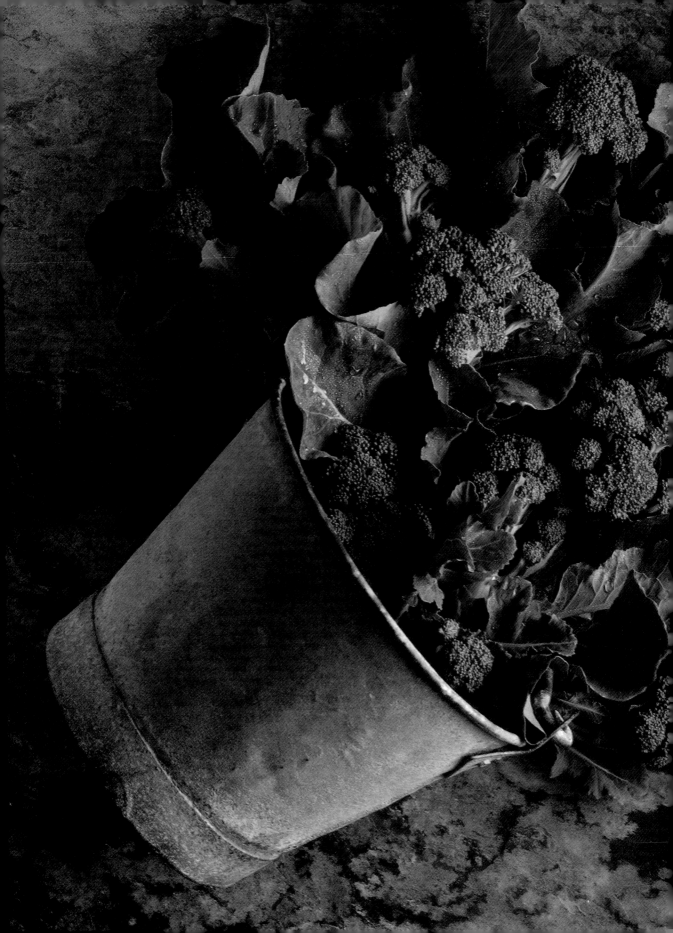

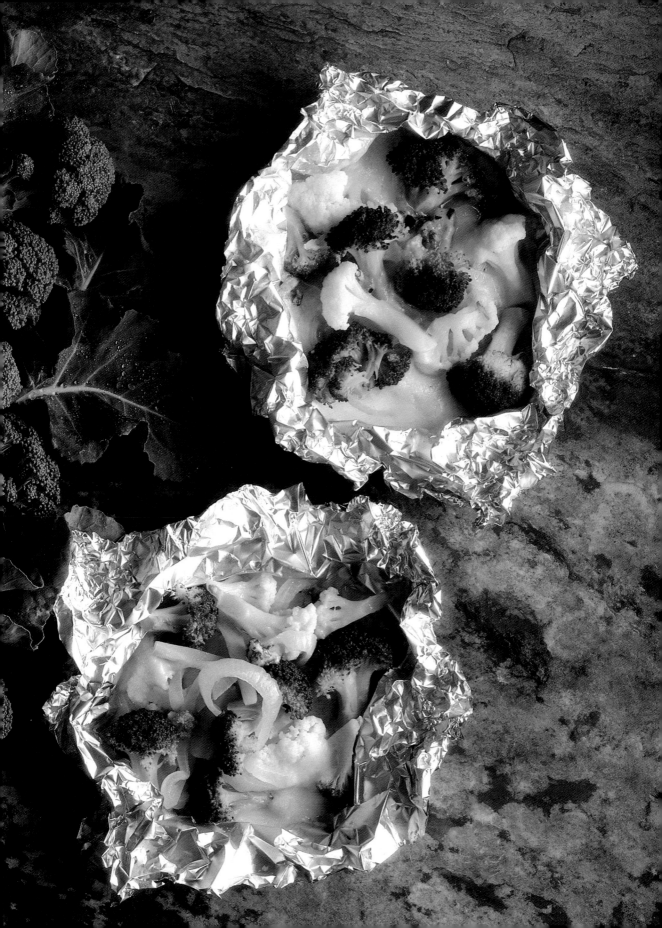

beaten egg and fold the pastry over the filling to form a half-circle pasty, pressing the edges firmly together and crimping. Lay on a baking tray and rest the pasties in the fridge for 30 minutes. Keep the remaining beaten egg.

Pre-heat the oven to gas mark 6, 400°F (200°C). Make a small hole in the centre of each pasty, then brush with the remaining beaten egg. Bake for 20–25 minutes until nicely browned. Serve hot, warm or cold.

Pasta with Broccoli, Ham and Gruyère

In the south of Italy, pasta and broccoli are cooked in the same pan, so that the pasta absorbs the flavour of the vegetable. It's a good method, even if the broccoli does end up a little battered in the process. I like to add two rather more northerly ingredients – ham and Gruyère – for extra oomph.

SERVES 4

450 g (1 lb) broccoli
450 g (1 lb) tagliatelle, fresh *or* dried
1 small onion, chopped
50 g (2 oz) butter
3 thick slices cooked ham, cut into strips
Salt and freshly ground black pepper
Ground nutmeg
100 g (4 oz) Gruyère cheese, grated

Separate the broccoli into small florets and slice the stems thinly.

Bring a large saucepan of lightly salted water to the boil. If using fresh pasta add the broccoli and 15 g (½ oz) butter, and simmer for 3 minutes. Add the tagliatelle, and bring back to the boil. Simmer until pasta is just *al dente*. Drain thoroughly and return to the pan. (For dried pasta add the tagliatelle to the saucepan at the same time as the broccoli and butter.)

Meanwhile, fry the onion in 25 g (1 oz) butter until tender, without browning. Add the ham and cook for a further 1–2 minutes. Turn the heat down low and keep warm. Once the pasta is drained and back in its pan, mix in the onion and ham and remaining butter, salt, pepper and nutmeg to taste. Quickly pile into a hot serving dish, and sprinkle with half the Gruyère. Serve immediately, with the remaining Gruyère for those who want it.

Cauliflower

Cauliflower, like broccoli, belongs to the same species as cabbage, *Brassica oleracea*. Gardeners may well shudder to hear that they belong to the botrytis group of this species. Happily, the name has nothing to do with the grey mildew, botrytis, that causes so much damage to vegetables. However, the two identical names are not entirely coincidental. Plants that are botryose bear flowers in clusters (the white curds of cauliflower are swollen clusters of flower buds). Botryoid, a word used in geology, means resembling clustered spheres. They all come from the Greek word *botrus*, meaning a bunch of grapes, and now we're getting close. The highly desirable 'noble rot' that settles on grapes, giving a honeyed stickiness to wines such as Sauternes, also takes its technical name from the Greek. It is *Botrytis cinerea*, not the same as, but related to common undesirable botrytis.

Whenever possible, buy cauliflowers that are still surrounded by a ruff of green leaves. The leaves are a better indication of freshness than the look of the white centre itself. If they are limp then the cauliflower has been away from the earth for far too long. The curd itself should be firm and creamy with a pleasant smell. Slight discoloration here and there is nothing to worry about. Always use cauliflower quickly, before it becomes stale.

Annabel's Cauliflower Salad

Annabel assists me in the kitchen, testing recipes, adjusting them so that they work, and often passing on her own good ideas. This salad is a favourite of hers, and rightly so. It's a lovely combination of flavours and textures, with that extra lift given by the horseradish.

SERVES 4–6

15 g (½ oz) flaked almonds
1 head of cauliflower, broken into small
    florets
8 tablespoons soured cream

1 tablespoon creamed horseradish
Squeeze of lemon juice
Salt and freshly ground black pepper
2 tablespoons chopped fresh chives

Pre-heat the oven to gas mark 6, 400°F (200°C). Spread the almonds out on a baking sheet and place in the oven for 3–7 minutes, shaking occasionally until golden brown. Cool.

Drop the cauliflower florets into a saucepan of lightly salted boiling water. Simmer until

OVERLEAF *Annabel's Cauliflower Salad*

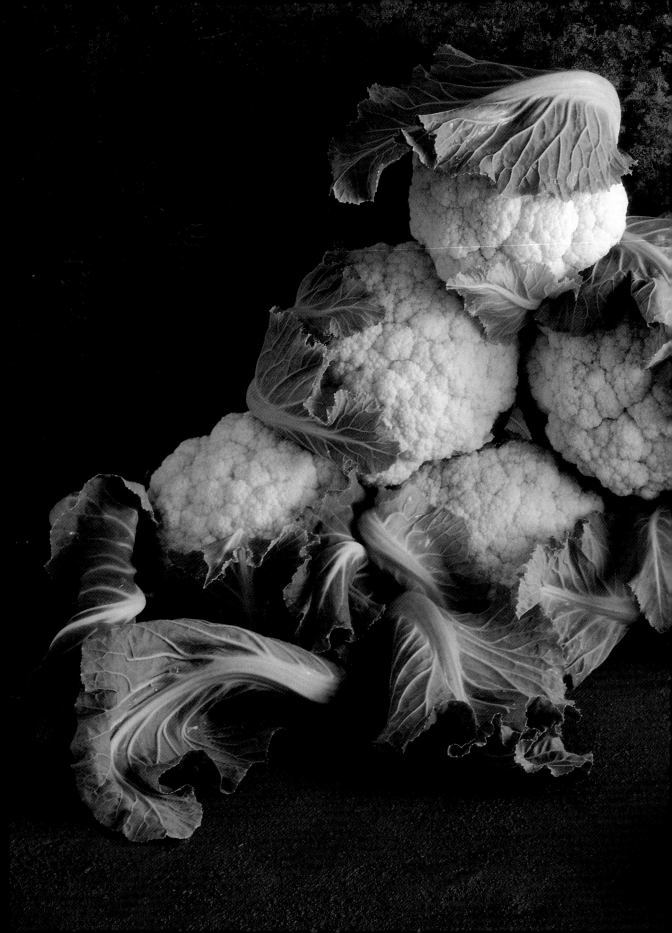

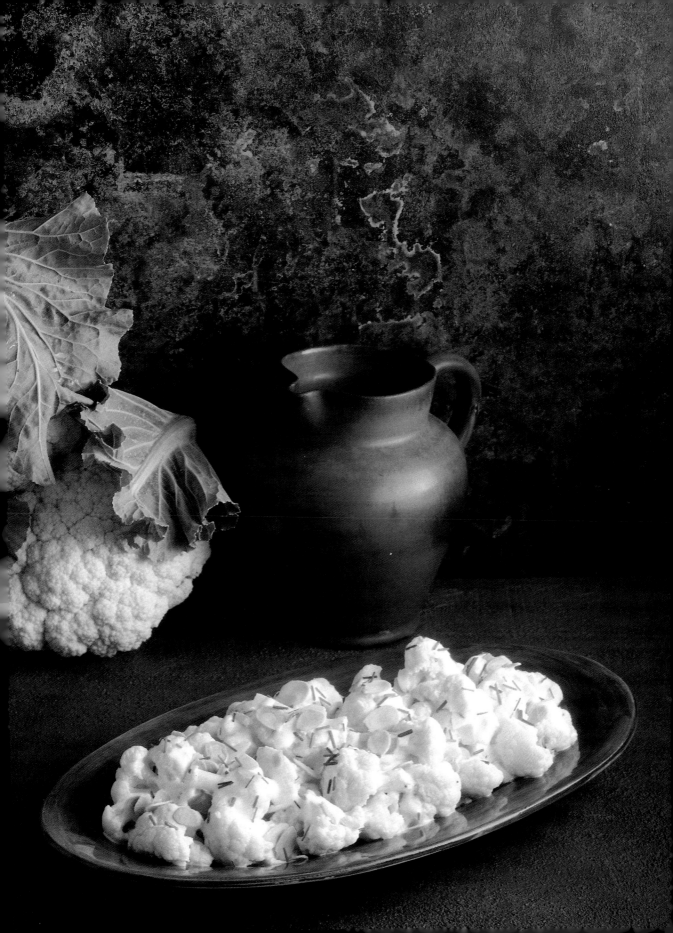

Preparing Cauliflower

To cook a whole cauliflower, trim off the leaves (which can be cooked as greens) and any small discoloured patches and make a deep criss-cross cut in the base so that it will cook more evenly. If you have a suitable metal basket, sit it in that and lower into a saucepan. Pour in enough boiling water to come about 7.5 cm (3 inches) up the cauliflower. Bring back to the boil, cover and simmer until just tender. Otherwise, make a 'cradle' by folding two long strips of silver foil in four lengthwise to strengthen them and then laying them out in a cross. Sit the cauliflower in the centre and bend the strips up and around it so that it can be lifted in and out of the pan safely. Either way, take special care not to overcook the cauliflower, or it will collapse as you transfer it to the dish.

I have mixed feelings about cauliflower as a vegetable. Boiled, particularly over-boiled, it is often singularly dull and it looks anaemic. Even perfectly cooked cauliflower needs a helping hand, something to inject a little vigour into its pallid soul.

School meals ruined cauliflower cheese for me, so I look for other ways to do the vegetable justice. When I'm going to serve it hot, I usually steam it until it is just tender but still with some firmness and resistance. Then I finish it by frying briefly in olive oil with garlic and adding a final sprinkling of parsley. I love it as a salad, too, again steamed, and tossed in vinaigrette and chopped herbs while still warm, or even nicer, finished with soured cream and almonds. Anchovies, chillies, cheese, crisp breadcrumbs, butter or good olive oil, spices and tomatoes are all great cauliflower improvers.

the cauliflower is barely *al dente* – just tender but with a slight crunch to it. Drain and run under the cold tap to prevent further cooking. Drain thoroughly and pat dry with kitchen paper.

Mix the soured cream with the horseradish, a dash of lemon juice, salt and pepper. Taste and adjust seasoning. Set aside a few of the almonds and chives to use as a garnish, then toss the remaining almonds, chives and cauliflower in the soured cream dressing. Arrange in a serving dish, and scatter with reserved almonds and chives. Serve at room temperature.

Parcels of Cauliflower and Broccoli Cheese

Wrapped up neatly in silver foil, these parcels of broccoli and cauliflower with two types of cheese are very handy for a dinner party. They can be prepared in advance, and whizzed into the oven, well out of the way, to get on with cooking all on their own. Serve the parcels unopened, so that each diner can have the pleasure of opening one for themselves.

SERVES 4

275–350 g (10–12 oz) broccoli
275–350 g (10–12 oz) cauliflower florets
1 onion, sliced
1 bay leaf
1 sprig of fresh thyme
 or ¼ teaspoon dried

1 sprig of fresh parsley
1 × 150-g (5-oz) ball of Mozzarella cheese, diced
75 g (3 oz) dolcelatte cheese, diced
Salt and freshly ground black pepper
2 tablespoons olive oil

Separate the stems and florets of broccoli. Cut the stems into 2.5-cm (1-inch) lengths. Place the stems in a saucepan with the cauliflower florets, onion, herbs, and enough salted water to cover by 1 cm (½ inch). Bring to the boil, add the broccoli florets and simmer for 1 minute. Drain and discard herbs. Cool the vegetables until tepid.

Pre-heat the oven to gas mark 4, 350°F (180°C). Mix vegetables carefully with Mozzarella and dolcelatte, pepper and a little salt. Take 4 large sheets of silver foil. Brush with a little oil, and mound up a quarter of the vegetable mixture on each sheet. Bring the sides up slightly around each one, and then drizzle ½ tablespoon of olive oil into each parcel.

Seal the parcels tightly, then sit on a baking tray. Bake for 30 minutes. Serve the parcels unopened.

Chilli-crumbed Cauliflower

Crisp-fried breadcrumbs with a hint of garlic and chilli are a quick way to liven up a dish of plain cooked cauliflower. A nice contrast, too, with the smoothness of the pale cauliflower.

SERVES 4–6

1 head of cauliflower, broken into florets
4 tablespoons olive oil
2 cloves garlic, peeled and finely chopped

1 green chilli, de-seeded and finely chopped
25 g (1 oz) fine white breadcrumbs
2 tablespoons chopped fresh parsley

Cook the cauliflower in salted boiling water, or steam. Drain well and arrange in a serving dish. Keep warm if necessary.

While the cauliflower is cooking heat the oil over a moderate heat and add the garlic, chilli and breadcrumbs. Fry until the crumbs are golden brown. Stir in the parsley, then immediately pour over the cauliflower and serve.

Dry Spiced Cauliflower

One of the best curries I had in India was, surprisingly enough, in the dingy restaurant in Delhi's small national airport. It was a dry cauliflower curry, scooped up with chapattis. Just as I was about to ask the man how it was made, our flight was called and we had to rush off. This is the best approximation to that curry that I've come up with yet. Not quite as it was, but a near thing.

SERVES 2 as a main course, 3–4 as a side dish

450 g (1 lb) cauliflower
2 tablespoons sunflower *or* vegetable oil
1-cm (½-inch) piece fresh ginger, peeled and finely chopped
2 cloves garlic, peeled and chopped
¼ teaspoon chilli powder
  or cayenne pepper

1 teaspoon ground turmeric
1½ teaspoons ground cumin
Salt
225 g (8 oz) tomatoes, skinned, de-seeded and chopped
1 teaspoon lemon juice
½ teaspoon garam masala (*optional*)

Break or cut the cauliflower into florets no larger than 2.5 cm (1 inch) long and wide.

Heat the oil in a frying-pan over a medium flame. Add the ginger and garlic and fry for about 30 seconds. Now add the chilli, turmeric and cumin. Stir and then add the cauliflower and salt. Turn gently so that the cauliflower is coated in spices, then add 4 tablespoons water. Turn the heat down low, and cover the pan tightly. Cook for 5 minutes.

Now add the tomatoes and lemon juice, stir to mix, and cover again. Cook for a further 5 minutes or so until the cauliflower is tender, stirring once. By the end of the cooking time, the vegetables should have absorbed virtually all the liquid. Sprinkle with garam masala, if using, and serve.

Cauliflower and Tomato Crumble

This recipe transforms cauliflower into a more substantial offering, with a savoury crumble topping that browns appetizingly in the heat of the oven. For a wetter dish, moisten the cauliflower in a bechamel sauce or tomato sauce before covering with the crumble mixture. Serve as a main, or first course.

SERVES 4–6

1 head of cauliflower, broken into florets
4 tomatoes, sliced

1 teaspoon fresh thyme leaves
  or ½ teaspoon dried
Salt and freshly ground black pepper
25 g (1 oz) butter

For the crumble
100 g (4 oz) plain flour
50 g (2 oz) rolled oats
50 g (2 oz) Cheddar cheese, grated

Salt and freshly ground black pepper
100 g (4 oz) butter

Cook the cauliflower in salted, boiling water, or steam, until almost tender. Pack tightly in a lightly buttered, heatproof dish. Cover with tomato slices. Sprinkle with thyme leaves, salt and pepper, then dot with the butter.

Pre-heat the oven to gas mark 6, 400°F (200°C).

To make the crumble, mix the flour, oats, grated cheese, salt and pepper together in a bowl. Melt the butter and stir enough of it into the mixture with a palette knife to make a crumbly mixture. Cool slightly then scatter over the vegetables in a thick layer. Bake for about 30 minutes until the crumble is golden brown and crisp. Serve immediately.

Chard

I first came across ruby chard in the glittering mosaicked food halls of Harrods. Though it wasn't in prime condition, its scarlet stems stood out like beacons. The dark leaves, veined with red, were floppy with age, but I bought it anyway. Who could resist such a beauty? Ruby or rhubarb chard, as the Americans call it, is a rarity in shops, but many gardeners grow it, often in amongst the flowers for a splash of bright colour. Since that first encounter, I've been lucky enough to cadge better, freshly picked specimens.

Ruby chard and the more familiar Swiss chard taste similar. Both are, effectively, two vegetables in one. The thick mid-ribs, pearly white or ruby red, are succulent and juicy, delicious steamed or boiled and served like asparagus with pools of melted butter. The leaves are more like a robust version of spinach and can be cooked in the same way. You could eat the mid-ribs as a first course and the leaves as a side dish with the main course.

Chard is much more popular on the continent than it is here. I've eaten squares of chard 'pizza' in Italy and Spain. In France it may go into blood puddings and other charcuterie items, soups and tarts. Sopas Mallorquinas is a warming thick chard, vegetable and bread stew from the Balearics, just the kind of thing I like on a cold night.

Sculptor Richard Logan, who grows a great deal of ruby chard on his allotment, as much for the colour as the taste, passed on a couple of ideas to me. He picks some of his crop when it is still young enough to eat raw in salads, a practical way of thinning out the plants so that they can mature to their full size and he also has an ingenious method for using the fully grown leaves. He substitutes them for the pasta when making lasagne.

Plain Cooked Chard

By sweating chard gently with nothing more than a few tablespoonfuls of olive oil for lubrication, you lose none of the flavour. Far better than boiling it when you want a fairly plain side dish.

SERVES 4

750 g–1 kg (1½–2 lb) Swiss
   or ruby chard
4 tablespoons olive oil

Salt and freshly ground black pepper
Squeeze of lemon juice

Preparing Chard

Usually, I cook the mid-ribs and leaves together, adding the leaves a few minutes after the ribs and sweating them both in butter or oil (see below). However, before they get into the pan, they need to be separated. I find that the easiest way is to pile 3 or 4 leaves up, and slice out the mid-ribs with a sharp knife. For a more perfect separation cut them individually with a knife or scissors. Pull any tough strings from the ribs as you cut them into suitable lengths.

The large leaves, blanched for seconds to render them supple, can also be used like vine leaves, as a wrapper for small parcels of food.

Separate the leaves from the thick ribs of the chard. Shred the leaves roughly. Slice ribs into 1-cm (½-inch) wide strips (across the stalk, not lengthways). Warm the oil in a wide frying-pan, and add the ribs. Stir to coat in oil, then cover and cook over a low heat, for about 10–15 minutes, stirring occasionally. Add the leaves, stir then cover again and cook for a further 5–10 minutes until all are tender. Season with salt and pepper and a squeeze of lemon juice. Serve.

Chard in a Curried Cream Sauce

This uses the same method as in the Plain cooked chard (see p. 231), but replaces the oil with butter, adds cream and curry powder – and you end up with a luxuriously rich way of presenting chard. Hopeless if you are watching the cholesterol, superb when you throw dietary cares to the wind.

SERVES 4

750 g–1 kg (1½–2 lb) Swiss *or* ruby chard	175 ml (6 fl oz) double cream
50 g (2 oz) butter	Salt and freshly ground black pepper
1 teaspoon mild curry powder	Squeeze of lemon juice

Separate the leaves from the thick ribs of the chard. Shred the leaves roughly. Slice ribs into 1-cm (½-inch) wide strips (across the stalk, not lengthways). Melt the butter in a wide frying-pan and add the ribs. Stir to coat in butter, then cover and cook over a low heat, for 10–15 minutes, stirring occasionally. Add the leaves and the curry powder, stir then cover again and cook for a further 5–10 minutes until all are tender. When the chard is done, pour over the cream and stir to mix. Simmer, uncovered for a few minutes until thickened, season with salt and pepper and a squeeze of lemon juice and serve.

Sopas Mallorquinas
[Mallorcan Vegetable and Bread Stew]

There are many different versions of Sopas Mallorquinas, but this is based on one I ate in Palma on my first trip to Mallorca. It is a sturdy peasant bread and vegetable stew, not elegant fare, but from the school of thrifty Mediterranean cooking that lets nothing to go to waste. Sopas does not, as one might fairly assume, mean soup. It is the name given to the thin dried slices of left-over bread that are used to soak up the juices of the vegetable broth. The final dish is not at all soupy, but thick and substantial. Sopas Mallorquinas tastes good made with plain water but even better with stock.

SERVES 4

150 g (5 oz) thin slices good bread
450 g (1 lb) Swiss chard
50 ml (2 fl oz) olive oil
4 cloves garlic, peeled and chopped
2 leeks, thinly sliced
450 g (1 lb) tomatoes, skinned and
    chopped

1 tablespoon chopped fresh marjoram
    or 1 teaspoon dried
1 tablespoon chopped fresh parsley
Salt and freshly-ground black pepper
300 ml (10 fl oz) water *or* stock
Extra virgin olive oil to serve

If you have the time, leave the bread out on an uncovered tray for several days until it is dried. Otherwise, spread the bread out on baking trays and bake in a very low oven (gas mark ½, 250°F, 120°C) until dry and brittle.

Cut the green parts off the Swiss chard and shred thinly. Save the ribs for another dish. Heat the olive oil in a wide deep frying-pan and add the garlic and leeks. Cook gently until tender, without browning. Add the tomatoes, marjoram and parsley and simmer until thickened. Add the shredded chard leaves, salt and pepper, water or stock and simmer until chard is tender. Taste and adjust seasonings.

Break up the slices of bread and place in a warmed bowl large enough to take the vegetable stew as well. When the stew is done, pour over the bread. Stir and let it stand for a few minutes so that the bread can soak up the juices, then trickle over a little extra olive oil and serve.

Swiss Chard with Olives au Gratin

I'm a sucker for gratins of any kind, bubbling and crustily brown, but the earthy taste of chard leaves, coupled with the juicy stalks and salty black olives make this an exceptionally good one.

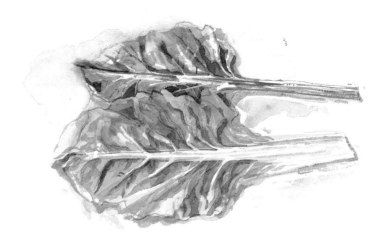

SERVES 4–6

750 g (1½ lb) Swiss chard *or* ruby chard
10 black olives, pitted and finely
    chopped
40 g (1½ oz) butter
½ small onion, chopped

25 g (1 oz) plain flour
300 ml (10 fl oz) milk
1 sprig of fresh thyme *or* pinch of dried
Salt and freshly ground black pepper
1 tablespoon grated Gruyère cheese

Pile up several chard leaves at a time and cut off the green leaves with scissors or a sharp knife. Cut the ribs into 4-cm (1½-inch) pieces, and shred the green parts finely. Steam or boil the ribs until tender, drain and spread in a 23-cm (9-inch) gratin dish. Scatter with the chopped olives.

Melt 15 g (½ oz) butter in a saucepan and add the shredded greenery and 2 tablespoons of water. Cover tightly and shake over a medium heat, stirring occasionally, until collapsed and tender. Cool slightly and squeeze out all the liquid. Chop roughly.

Melt the remaining butter in a small saucepan, and fry the onion gently until tender. Sprinkle with the flour and cook for a minute. Off the heat, add the milk gradually to make a white sauce. Return to the heat, add the thyme and simmer for a good 5 minutes. Remove the thyme stalk, stir in the cooked greenery, a little salt and plenty of pepper. Spoon over the chard stems and sprinkle with the grated Gruyère. If all the ingredients are still hot, just whip under the grill to brown. Otherwise, bake at gas mark 6, 400°F (200°C) for 20 minutes until browned and bubbling. Serve immediately.

PODS and SEEDS

Peas • French Beans (Green Beans)
Broad Beans • Sweetcorn • Okra

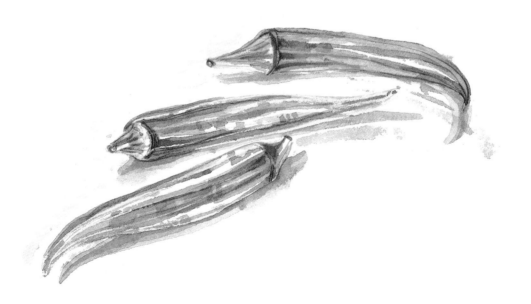

Peas

I eat my peas with honey,
I've done it all my life.
They taste a little bit funny,
But it makes them stick on the knife.

Actually, I don't eat my peas with honey – peas are quite sweet enough as they are – but the rhyme dances through my head whenever I cook peas. Like most people, most of the time, I resort to frozen peas, but it's a case of second-best. Fresh peas picked straight from the garden and cooked within a couple of hours eclipse convenience peas with ease. The difference is astounding. The everyday pea becomes an item of incomparable luxury.

Shop-bought peas in their pods lie somewhere between truly fresh and frozen in value. They've often been hanging around for several days and their fresh flavour is diminished. If you don't grow your own, my advice is to make friends with someone who does then at least you may be invited to share their treasure once in a while.

Garden peas can be so sweet and tender that one is tempted not to cook them at all. Wandering through the immaculately neat allotment of 15-year-old David Johnson, we pulled peas from the vine and ate them straight out of the pod as we talked. Gifted with green fingers, he's grown plants of one kind or another ever since he can remember. He acquired his allotment when he was 12, and his rows of bushy pea plants, almost over-burdened with their heavy crop of pods, are his pride and joy. I found it hard to tear myself away, finally grabbing a couple of pods to take with me on my journey home. David insists that peas are not difficult to grow. If only I had the space in my small garden . . .

Pea, Ricotta and Herb Quiche

This is an enchantingly pretty, country-ish quiche, with a puffed yeast dough crust, filled with herb-flecked ricotta and peas. I think that the yeast pastry is what makes it extra special, but if you are pushed for time, line the tart tin with shortcrust pastry (see p. 20) and bake blind before filling. Use a mixture of at least three sweet, fresh herbs, such as parsley, chives, chervil, basil or marjoram. Thyme, lovage or salad burnet are good too, but use in comparatively small quantities as they are strongly flavoured. Like most quiches, this one tastes nicest when served warm.

SERVES 6–8

For the pastry

200 g (7 oz) strong white bread flour
½ packet easybake
   or easyblend dried yeast

Salt
1 egg
3 tablespoons olive oil

For the filling

225 g (8 oz) ricotta
2 eggs
200 ml (7 fl oz) milk
4 tablespoons freshly grated Parmesan
   cheese
4 spring onions, thinly sliced

3 tablespoons chopped mixed sweet
   fresh herbs (e.g. parsley, chives,
   chervil, basil, marjoram, oregano,
   thyme, lovage, salad burnet)
Salt and freshly ground black pepper
350 g (12 oz) cooked peas

Sift the flour with the salt. Stir in the yeast. Make a well in the centre and break in the egg. Add the oil. Gradually work into the flour, adding enough water to form a soft dough. (Use a food processor for maximum speed and ease.) Gather the dough up into a ball, knead for 5–10 minutes until smooth and elastic, set in a clean bowl, cover and leave to rise in a warm place until it has doubled in bulk.

While it rises, prepare the filling. Beat the ricotta with the eggs, and gradually mix in the milk. Stir in 3 tablespoons of the Parmesan, and all the spring onions, herbs, salt and pepper.

Place an upturned metal baking sheet in the oven, and heat to gas mark 5, 375°F (190°C). Punch down the dough and knead again briefly. Using the heel of your hand, press the dough into an oiled 25-cm (10-inch) tart tin, easing the dough to cover the base and come up around the sides. The dough should be thickest around the sides, rising up a little above the rim of the tin.

Scatter the peas evenly over the dough. Stir the ricotta custard and pour over the peas. Sprinkle the remaining tablespoon of Parmesan over the surface. Set on the hot baking sheet in the oven (which gives the base of the tart an instant blast of heat) and bake for 30–35 minutes until barely set and golden. Serve hot, warm or cold.

OVERLEAF *Pea, Ricotta and Herb Quiche*

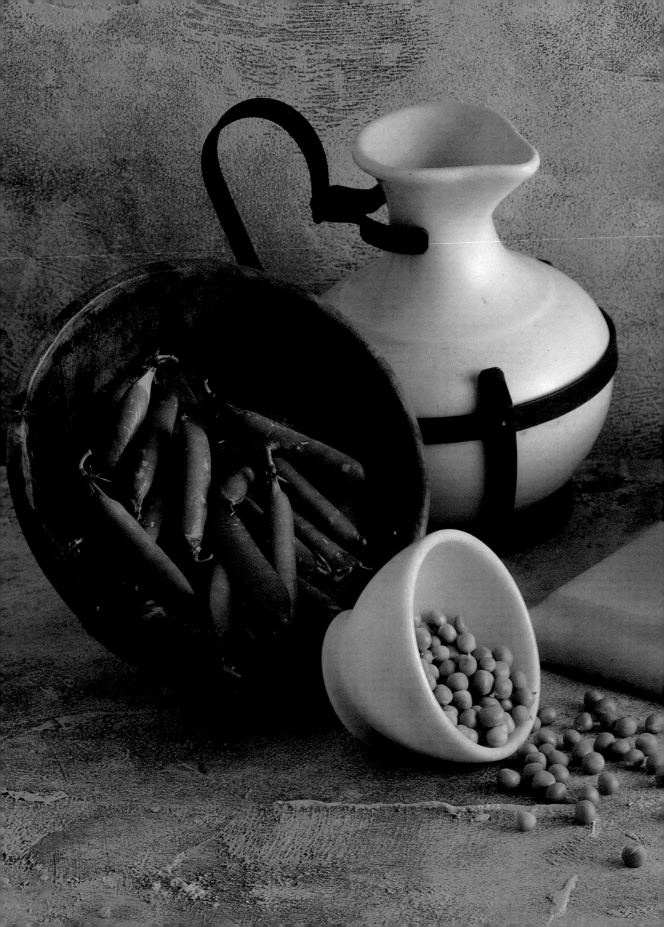

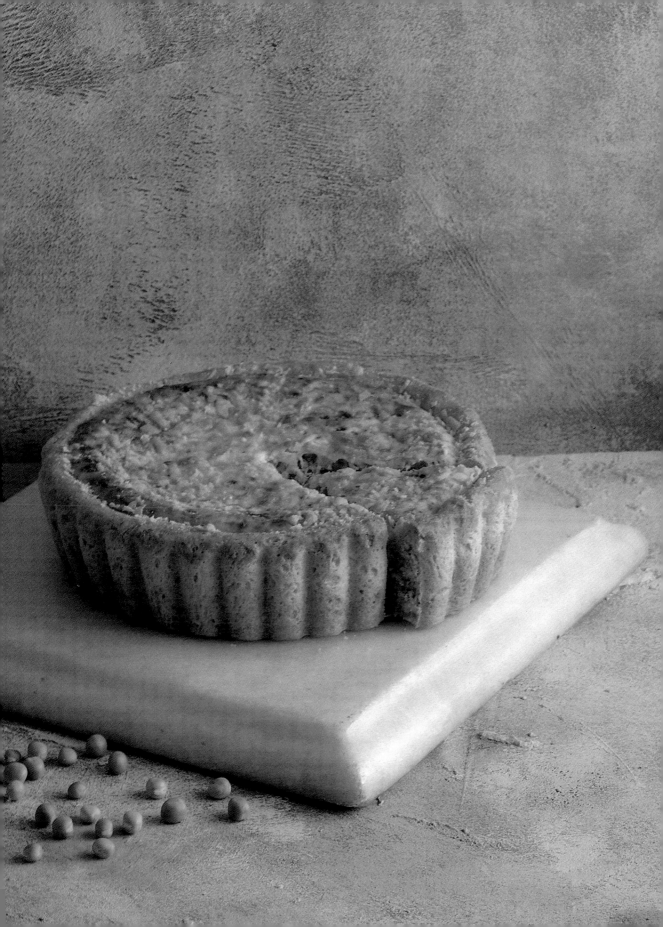

Preparing Peas

The traditional British way of cooking peas with sprigs of fresh mint is one of the best. Some people add a pinch of sugar too, but it's quite unnecessary with newly picked garden peas or frozen peas. It does help shop-bought fresh peas regain some of their natural sweetness. Pea pods shouldn't be wasted. Chopped up, they make a good soup (sieve it to remove the tough strings). If you grow your own peas, try picking them on the small side and cooking them whole, to serve as a course on their own with plenty of butter. To eat, pick them up with the fingers and draw out the peas and the soft flesh of the pods with your teeth.

Peas make good ingredients in composite dishes, both for their taste and their bright colour. For example, they are essential to a Navarin printanier (see p. 242), *the* springtime stew, and make a good addition to other stews too. When I use frozen peas for these kinds of dishes, I thaw them first so that they don't instantly lower the temperature in the pan when they are added. If I've forgotten to take them from the freezer in time to thaw naturally, I break up the frozen clumps, then cover with boiling water which soon takes the chill off. Frozen peas have already been cooked, so should be added towards the end of the cooking time. Incidentally, I always find the cooking time given on the packet far too long. They taste best boiled for a few minutes, just long enough to heat through.

To be frank, I've gotten a little bored with mangetout peas. They've been over-exposed, and too often overcooked into the bargain. I do still add them, raw, to salads (topped and tailed first), and occasionally use them in stir-fries where they retain a good deal of their crispness. Steamed or boiled, mangetout peas need only 3 or 4 minutes, just time to soften without becoming soggy and insubstantial.

I far prefer sugarsnap peas, which marry the best of mangetout and ordinary peas. Plump and filled with proper little peas, they are tender enough to eat whole. Like mangetouts, they are good raw in salads, but even nicer steamed.

Guisantes con Jamon
[Peas with Ham]

This Spanish way of cooking peas highlights their natural sweetness with the saltiness of cured jamon serrano, the superb dried mountain ham. If you don't have a Spanish supplier near you, Parma ham makes a good substitute. Normally, I wouldn't cook frozen peas for 30−40 minutes, but in this recipe they need time to absorb the flavour of the ham.

SERVES 4

1 kg (2 lb) peas in their pods	2 tablespoons olive oil
or 450 g (1 lb) thawed, frozen peas	50–75-g (2–3-oz) piece Spanish jamon
1 carrot, peeled and very finely chopped	serrano *or* other dried raw ham
1 onion, finely chopped	Sweet paprika to garnish

Shell the fresh peas, if using. In a saucepan large enough to hold the peas in a layer no more than 2.5 cm (1 inch) thick, sauté the carrot and onion in the oil until the onion is golden brown. Add the ham, and stir for a further 30 seconds or so, then add the peas. Stir, then cover tightly and cook slowly for 30–40 minutes, until the peas are tender (if using frozen peas reduce the cooking time by 10 minutes). Stir occasionally, to make sure that they don't catch on the base. Dust with paprika before serving.

Risi e Bisi
[Rice and Peas]

This is a Venetian dish. Though the peas and rice are cooked together in one large pot, it's not a risotto. In fact, it requires much less effort, as there is no need to stir constantly as it cooks. The result is soupier, and lacks the creaminess of a risotto, but it is, nonetheless, quite delicious.

SERVES 4

450 g (1 lb) peas in their pods	1 onion, chopped
or 225 g (8 oz) shelled peas, fresh	4 tablespoons chopped fresh parsley
or frozen	200 g (7 oz) Arborio rice
1.2 litres (2 pints) chicken stock	3 tablespoons freshly grated Parmesan
50 g (2 oz) butter	cheese
2 tablespoons olive oil	Salt and freshly ground black pepper
50 g (2 oz) pancetta *or* cured raw ham	Extra freshly grated Parmesan cheese to
(e.g. Parma ham), chopped	serve

Shell the peas if using peas in their pods. Put the stock in a saucepan and bring gently to the boil. Meanwhile, prepare the 'sofrito' – heat half the butter and all the oil in a large saucepan. Add the pancetta or ham, onion, and parsley. Cook over a gentle heat until the onions are tender, without browning. Add the peas, and stir for a few minutes.

Now add the hot stock and bring back to the boil. Pour in the rice in a steady stream, then season with salt and pepper. Simmer for about 15–20 minutes until the rice is just tender. Draw off the heat and stir in the remaining butter and the Parmesan cheese.

Serve in deep bowls, passing round extra Parmesan for those who want it.

Duck Stewed with Green Peas

Duck stewed with green peas is generally accepted as a classic of the English kitchen, though in fact it's a combination that originated in France. I've tried several versions, but come back, time and again to the eighteenth-century recipe that my mother, Jane Grigson, gave in her Vegetable Book.

SERVES 4

2 sprigs of fresh parsley
1 bay leaf
2 sprigs of fresh thyme
1 large sprig of fresh rosemary
1 large duck
Oil for browning
300 ml (10 fl oz) duck giblet stock
  or game stock *or* well-flavoured
  chicken stock

1 large, crisp lettuce, shredded
450 g (1 lb) shelled peas
Salt and freshly ground black pepper
2 egg yolks
5 tablespoons double cream
Squeeze of lemon juice

Tuck all the herbs inside the duck. Prick the skin all over with a fork. Brown the duck briskly in a little oil in a large flameproof casserole or heavy saucepan. Pour off any excess fat, and settle the duck breast-side down in the casserole, adding the stock. Cover and simmer for 1¼ hours.

Turn the duck upright, stuff the shredded lettuce down around it, and add the peas, salt and pepper. Cover again, and simmer for a further 45 minutes.

Lift out the duck and keep warm on a serving dish. Scoop out the vegetables and arrange around it. Skim off the fat from the cooking liquid in the pot. Beat the egg yolks and cream together and stir into the juices, keeping the heat low so that the sauce thickens without curdling – don't let it get anywhere near boiling point. Season and add lemon juice to taste. Serve with the duck.

Navarin Printanier
[Springtime Lamb and Vegetable Casserole]

Made in spring, with small succulent vegetables, a Navarin printanier is a real treat. I make it to celebrate the end of winter, as a personal signal that summer is on the way, even if there is still a nip in the air. Later on in the year, use larger potatoes, carrots and turnips cut into cubes to make a Navarin, minus the Printanier (it means spring in the adjectival sense, so would be quite inappropriate in, say, September), but don't expect the flavour to be quite so fine.

SERVES 6

1.5 kg (3 lb) shoulder of lamb, trimmed
    and cubed
25 g (1 oz) butter
1 tablespoon sunflower oil
2 tablespoons plain flour
1 pint lamb, light chicken
    or vegetable stock
1 tablespoon tomato purée

Bouquet garni (see p. 36)
1 clove garlic, peeled and crushed
Salt and freshly ground black pepper
450 g (1 lb) new potatoes, scrubbed
225 g (8 oz) small carrots
225 g (8 oz) small turnips, peeled
350 g (12 oz) shelled peas

Brown the lamb in the butter and oil over a high heat, in several batches so as not to overcrowd the frying-pan. Transfer the lamb to a heatproof casserole and pour off all except about 2 tablespoons of the fat left in the frying-pan. Add the flour and stir over a moderate heat until you have a light brown roux. Stir in the stock gradually, and then the tomato purée. Bring to the boil, then pour over the meat. Add the bouquet garni, garlic and salt and pepper. Cover and simmer very gently for about 1 hour.

Then add the potatoes, carrots and turnips and continue simmering very gently, still covered, for a further 40 minutes. If necessary, add a little more water or stock as it cooks – you are aiming to end up with a creamy, but not thick, sauce about the consistency of single cream. Now add the peas and continue cooking until all the vegetables are tender. Taste and adjust seasoning. Serve.

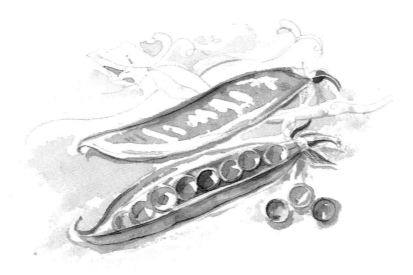

French Beans (Green Beans)

The Reverend Mervyn Wilson's garden seems a million miles away from the twentieth century. It's a haven of tranquillity, mysterious and romantic with its long vistas between high yew hedges to the dovecot, the hidden bench under a medlar tree, an alley of apple trees leading to the belvedere, and old roses climbing and tumbling through plum trees.

The kitchen garden is tucked away, more orderly than the rest of the garden with neat rows of greenery. Here, Reverend Wilson has gathered together a fine collection of beans of different types. Naturally, there are scarlet runners and climbing green French beans, but he also grows a late-maturing type of French bean known as Marvel of Venice (which has the best flavour of all, he says), purple skinned climbing beans, old fashioned red-and-white beans, dwarf green and purple French beans and yellow wax beans . . . I'd never seen such a number of varieties massed together on one small site. The Reverend Wilson, complete with dog-collar, wellington boots, and wooden trug, picked a bagful of beans of all hues for me to take home and compare.

French beans or string beans, as Americans call them, are a type of immature kidney bean. If they were left to grow on the plant to their full size, the pod or 'haulm' would stretch and dry to a papery parchment enclosing the swelling semi-dried seeds inside. The fully formed seeds can be eaten straight from the plant, simply boiled and served with butter, or dried and stored for winter use.

Purple French beans look very dramatic as they dangle amongst the leaves – easy to see and easy to harvest. Though they taste good, they are a disappointment – like so many dark, purple-black vegetables, the colour reverts to green when cooked. I prefer the yellow wax beans which keep their colour and have a buttery taste and smooth texture.

Unless you grow these coloured varieties or have an enterprising local greengrocer, familiar green beans are probably all you'll be able to lay your hands on. 'Dwarf beans' and 'Kenyan beans' are slightly chunkier types of French bean, not quite as refined as thinner French beans.

Preparing French Beans

Whatever variety or colour of French bean you are using, they are all prepared and cooked in the same way. Always choose beans that are stiff and firm – floppy limpness is an unmistakable steer clear signal. To prepare, just top and tail, pulling off any strings as you work (unless they are very small in which case there's no need to bother). If I'm in a hurry and have a big heap of beans to deal with, I gather them into bundles and slice the ends off. The one problem with this method is that any strings are left in place, but most modern varieties are bred to be as string-free as possible, so with luck this will mean only a rare moment of unwanted chewing.

Whether you steam or boil French beans, don't overdo it. Flabby beans are boring. They should be tender enough, but still slightly firm in the centre. Between 5 and 10 minutes depending on thickness is all it will take. If you boil them, keep the lid off to preserve their vivid colour. Cooked beans are lovely in salads, tossed while still warm in a vinaigrette or the anchovy dressing on p. 178, or with bacon and Worcestershire sauce (see below).

French Bean and Bacon Salad

Once a year I teach a children's cookery holiday, and on the last day the children and I have to prepare a meal for 70 people between us. We use whatever vegetables we have to hand to make huge bowls of salad. I gave one group of boys a box of French beans and some bacon, a few vague instructions, and this was what they came up with, though in rather larger quantity. The garlic and Worcestershire sauce were their additions, and are what really make the salad.

SERVES 4

450 g (1 lb) French beans
4 rashers streaky bacon
2 tablespoons chopped fresh parsley

For the dressing
1 clove garlic, peeled and crushed
½ tablespoon white wine vinegar
1 teaspoon Worcestershire sauce
3 tablespoons olive oil
Salt and freshly ground black pepper

To make the dressing, whisk the crushed garlic with the vinegar and Worcestershire sauce. Gradually beat in the olive oil, and add salt and pepper to taste.

Top and tail the beans and cut into 2.5–4-cm (1–1½-inch) lengths. Drop into a pan of boiling salted water and simmer for about 3 minutes or until just tender but retaining a slight crunch. Drain thoroughly and mix with enough of the dressing to coat well. Grill the rashers of bacon until browned then cut into small strips. Toss with the green beans and the parsley. Taste, and adjust seasoning, adding a little extra Worcestershire sauce if necessary. Serve.

French Beans with Cumin and Almonds

Who would have thought that adding a spoonful of cumin and a few almonds to a panful of French beans would turn them into something so exotic? Well, it does, though they're not so over-the-top exotic as to clash with an otherwise straightforward meal.

SERVES 4

450 g (1 lb) French beans, topped and tailed
2 tablespoons olive *or* sunflower oil *or* 25 g (1 oz) butter

15 g (½ oz) flaked almonds
1 small onion, chopped
1 teaspoon ground cumin
Salt and freshly ground black pepper

Cut the beans into 2.5–4-cm (1–1½-inch) lengths.

Heat the oil or butter in a wide frying-pan. Fry the almonds briskly until golden brown. Scoop out and drain on kitchen paper. Reduce the heat under the pan and fry the onions until tender, without browning. Add the beans, cumin and salt and pepper and fry for 3 minutes. Add 2 tablespoons of water, then cover and cook for 5 minutes or so until the beans are tender and most of the liquid has been absorbed. Return the almonds to the pan, stir for a few seconds to re-heat, and serve.

Curried Beans à la Crème

This curried cream sauce is much the same as the one I use for chard (see p. 232), but the final dishes taste quite different. Instead of the dark savouriness of the chard, it is the sweet snap of French beans that picks up the mild fragrance of curry.

SERVES 4

450 g (1 lb) green (French) beans, topped and tailed
25 g (1 oz) butter
1 teaspoon mild curry powder

120 ml (4 fl oz) whipping cream
Salt and freshly ground black pepper
Dash of lemon juice

Cut the beans in half, and blanch in boiling salted water for 3–4 minutes. Drain thoroughly.

Melt the butter in a wide frying-pan. When it is foaming, add the beans and fry for 1 minute. Sprinkle over the curry powder and mix in, then fry for a further minute. Add the cream and a little salt and pepper and simmer until the cream has reduced to a thick sauce. Draw off the heat and add a squeeze of lemon juice to highlight the flavours. Taste and adjust seasoning and serve.

Bean and Potato Ratatouille

This isn't a ratatouille in the real sense of the word, but the cooking method is similar, even if French beans and potatoes do replace the aubergines, courgettes and peppers. In fact, the dill gives it more of an Eastern Mediterranean flavour. Like ratatouille, it can be served hot or cold, as a side dish, first course or even a main course, perhaps with a few eggs poached in it when it is nearly done.

SERVES 4–6

1 onion, chopped
2 cloves garlic, peeled and chopped
4 tablespoons extra virgin olive oil
275 g (10 oz) new potatoes *or* waxy salad
  potatoes, halved or quartered if large
750 g (1½ lb) fresh tomatoes, skinned,
  de-seeded and chopped
  or 1½ × 400 g (14 oz) tins
  chopped tomatoes

1 tablespoon tomato purée
½ tablespoon sugar
Salt and freshly ground black pepper
350 g (12 oz) French beans, topped and
  tailed and cut in half
2 tablespoons chopped fresh parsley
1½ tablespoons chopped fresh dill
  or ½ tablespoon dried

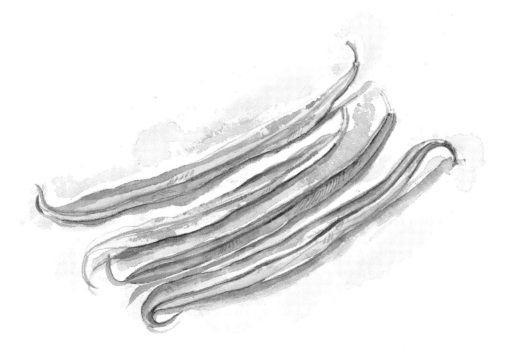

Cook the onion and garlic gently in 3 tablespoons of the oil in a large saucepan until tender, without browning. Add the potatoes, stir, then cover and cook for a further 5 minutes. Add the tomatoes, tomato purée, sugar, salt and pepper. Bring to the boil and simmer, uncovered, until the potatoes are half-cooked.

Put in the beans, 1 tablespoon of the parsley and all the dill. Simmer for a further 10–15 minutes, stirring occasionally, until the vegetables are all tender and the sauce is thick. If the sauce still looks a bit watery, turn up the heat and boil hard for a few minutes to reduce. Taste and adjust seasonings. Serve hot or cold and, just before serving, sprinkle with remaining parsley and drizzle the last tablespoon of olive oil over the 'ratatouille'.

Sichuan Green Beans

This recipe first appeared in my earlier book, Sophie's Table, *but there was no way I could leave it out of this chapter on green beans. It is just too good and too remarkable. Until I came across it, it had never occurred to me to deep-fry green beans. In fact, it is an excellent way of cooking them, even if you don't go on to finish them with all the aromatics. However, I'd urge you to try the full treatment. Dried shrimps and Sichuan pepper can be found in Chinese food shops.*

SERVES 4 as a first course

2 tablespoons dried shrimps
½ kg (1 lb) French beans, topped and
    tailed
Sunflower or vegetable oil for
    deep-frying
2 cloves garlic, peeled and thinly sliced
½ teaspoon Sichuan *or* black pepper-
    corns, coarsely crushed

2.5-cm (1-inch) piece of fresh ginger,
    peeled and cut into matchsticks
½ teaspoon salt
1 tablespoon sugar
1 tablespoon dark soy sauce
2 teaspoons rice vinegar
    or white wine vinegar
1 tablespoon sesame oil

Cover the shrimps generously with boiling water and soak for 20 minutes. Drain and reserve the liquid. Chop the shrimps finely. Heat a panful of oil to 190°C/375°F and deep-fry the beans for 5 minutes, until tender and patched with brown. Drain on kitchen paper.

In a wok, or large high-sided frying-pan, heat 1 tablespoon of oil until it smokes. Add the garlic, pepper and ginger and stir-fry for a few seconds. Then add the shrimps and stir-fry for 30 seconds. Add the salt, sugar, soy sauce and 5 tablespoons of the shrimp water.

Finally add the green beans. Toss in the sauce to coat well, then cover and, keeping the heat high, cook until virtually all the liquid has been absorbed. Check after 1 minute – the sauce should have caramelized and the beans should be several shades darker, even verging on black. Toss and, if necessary, cover again for a further 30 seconds or so to finish cooking. Remove from the heat and mix with the rice vinegar and sesame oil. Serve hot, or better still, cold.

Broad Beans

our of the leading families of ancient Rome had leguminous names. Most renowned was Cicero of the chickpea family, but there was also Piso, after peas, Lentulus, after lentils, and Fabius, after fava or faba beans or in other words, broad beans. There's a fact we were never taught at school. A shame – it might have given us a whole new perspective on Roman culture and colonization.

I've yet to find an explanation as to how or why these families got their names, but one thing it does indicate is that legumes have long played an important role in Europe – our modern broad bean is a direct but improved descendant of the field bean that has been cultivated since Stone Age times.

Their popularity amongst gardeners remains undimmed. I've seen many a clump of broad bean plants tucked away in gardens with otherwise fairly negligible vegetable plots. They are an immensely rewarding plant to grow, thriving on poor soil with little attention and yielding a generous crop. Then there is the pleasure afforded by the first, young tender beans of the early sumer. It's a shame that only gardeners and their friends can enjoy them at their best, before they mature to the coarse size of shop-bought broad beans.

When they are very small, no more than 75 cm (3 inches) in length, you can eat the entire pod, cooked like sugarsnap peas in boiling water and served with a knob of butter. At this stage they are fiddly to shell, but worth it for the succulent little beans, tender enough to eat raw with cured ham or cheese and bread as a simple, earthy treat.

Those of us who do not have a clump of broad bean plants have to make do with larger beans and though they may not be quite so special, they can still be delicious given the right treatment.

I'm well aware of the fact that many people loathe broad beans. It's the tough grey outer skin that is the culprit, imparting a coarse flavour and texture and getting irritatingly stuck between the teeth. Take the time to remove the skin and broad beans are transformed into a completely new vegetable, like a butterfly emerging from a chrysalis. The inner beanlets have a brilliant green colour, a vivid flavour and a marvellous mealy softness.

Preparing Broad Beans

Skinning individual beans is easy, but not a task to be undertaken when you are in a hurry to get supper on the table. Still, if you do have the time, it is worth every minute spent on it. To skin fresh, shelled broad beans, drop them into a pan of boiling water and blanch for 1 minute. Drain, run under the cold tap, then slit the skin of each bean and squeeze out the beanlet inside. To skin frozen broad beans (broad beans freeze very well though they will never be as good as freshly picked), either let them thaw out, or place in a bowl and cover with boiling water, leaving for a minute or so before draining. Then the skins will slip off easily. Once skinned return the beanlets to boiling salted water and finish cooking. Fresh ones will need only 5 minutes or so, frozen ones even less time.

Plainly cooked, skinned beans, served with a knob of butter are delightful, but you could finish the cooking by braising them gently with butter, a couple of tablespoonfuls of water and a few sprigs of savory – the herb always used by the French with broad beans – or thyme, in a covered pan for an even better result. I have a particular passion for broad bean purées – both the one in this section (see p. 253), and the garlic-scented one on p. 109. I like them, too, in salads, quiches and soups. About the one thing I can't take, is tough broad beans in gluey white sauce – a dismal ending for a vegetable with such a distinguished ancestry.

As a rough guide 1.5 kg (3 lb) of fresh broad beans in their pods will yield around 450 g (1 lb) of shelled beans.

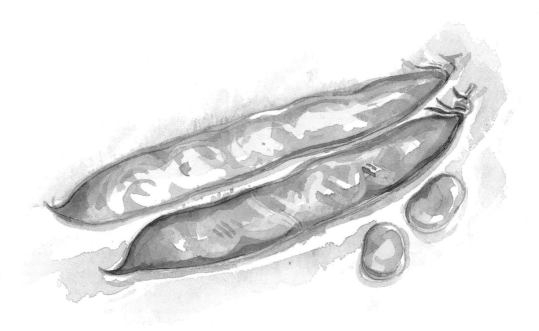

Brigid Allen's Broad Bean Soup with Pesto

Brigid Allen was brought up thinking that soup was pretty dull stuff. Then, during a stay at a convent in France, the nuns served up a delicious, home-made, fresh celery soup, flavoured with chervil. For Brigid it was a blinding moment of revelation. A few years later she tasted her first real minestrone in Italy which finally set her on the path towards a true passion for soup. Her experiments with combinations of ingredients have culminated in a book called The Soup Book *(Papermac) in which the following two recipes appear. As far as possible she uses fresh ingredients from her garden, as she does for this delicious broad bean soup. Totally uncompromising where her recipes are concerned, Brigid highly disapproves of shop-bought pesto and always makes her own, occasionally substituting cashew nuts for the more traditional pinenuts. She would certainly never use frozen broad beans. However, if you do resort to the freezer, thaw the beans before adding them to the soup.*

SERVES 4

2 onions, chopped
2 carrots, peeled and diced
2 tablespoons olive oil

For the pesto
4–5 cloves garlic, peeled
12–15 large leaves fresh basil
40 g (1½ oz) pinenuts
  or broken cashew nuts

1 kg (2 lb) broad beans, shelled
  or 450 g (1 lb) shelled weight
1.5 litres (2½ pints) water
1 teaspoon sea salt

40 g (1½ oz) freshly grated Parmesan
  cheese
Sea salt
3–4 tablespoons extra virgin olive oil

Put the onions, carrots and olive oil in a pan, stir, then cover and cook over a low heat for 10–15 minutes. Add the shelled beans, cover and cook for 1–2 minutes more. Cover with the water and add the salt. Bring to the boil and simmer for 20 minutes.

Meanwhile, make the pesto. If you have a food processor that can handle small quantities, whizz the garlic, basil, nuts and cheese together with a pinch of salt, gradually drizzling in the olive oil. Otherwise, use a large mortar or a small pudding basin wedged so that it will not skid. Crush the garlic with a pinch of sea salt, add the basil leaves and pound them into the garlic until you have an aromatic, green sludge. Add the nuts and grind them into the mixture until they have merged with the basil and garlic. Stir in the grated cheese and enough olive oil to give a loose, but not runny, mixture.

Liquidize the soup and re-heat if necessary. Taste and adjust the seasonings. Stir in the pesto just before serving.

Brigid Allen's Green Velvet Soup

This thick, dark green soup with its subtle, intriguing taste is the result of Brigid's experiments with tops pinched out from her broad bean plants also good in salads when lightly cooked. The shoyu and tamari she uses are Japanese forms of soy sauce with a particularly full flavour.

SERVES 4

2 onions, chopped
2 tablespoons sunflower oil
2 courgettes, sliced
225 g (8 oz) broad bean tops

1.5 litres (2½ pints) chicken stock
or 1.5 litres (2½ pints) water and
1–2 tablespoons shoyu (or tamari)
Sea salt
2 handfuls of sorrel, shredded (*optional*)

Cook the onion in the oil in a heavy, covered pan over a low heat for 10 minutes. Add the courgettes, stir, then cook over a low to moderate heat for another 5–10 minutes, stirring every now and then to make sure that they do not brown.

Meanwhile, wash the bean tops, carefully checking for signs of blackfly, and add them to the pan. Cover with the stock or water and add salt. Bring to the boil and simmer for 20 minutes. A few minutes before the end of cooking, add the sorrel if using. Liquidize and re-heat if necessary, stirring in shoyu or tamari to taste if water was used instead of stock.

Broad Bean, Red Pepper and Courgette Salad

This is a gloriously summery salad for when the first broad beans are ready to be harvested. It looks pretty and light-hearted – red and green dotted with black olives.

SERVES 4–6

450 g (1 lb) small courgettes
1 red pepper

350 g (12 oz) shelled broad beans
10 black olives, pitted and halved

For the dressing

1 tablespoon balsamic *or* sherry vinegar
or red wine vinegar *or* 1½ tablespoons lemon juice
Salt and freshly ground black pepper

4–6 tablespoons extra virgin olive oil
½ tablespoon chopped fresh tarragon *or*
1 tablespoon mixed finely chopped
fresh parsley and fresh chervil

First make the dressing. Whisk the vinegar or lemon juice with salt and pepper, and gradually whisk in the oil a tablespoon at a time. Add the herbs. Taste and adjust seasonings.

Grill and skin the pepper (see p. 168). Cut into strips. Turn in a little of the dressing to keep moist. Cook the broad beans in salted boiling water, drain, then run under the cold tap. Slip the inner beans out of the coarse grey skins if you have time, then toss the beans in a little of the dressing.

Steam or boil the courgettes until just *al dente*. Drain thoroughly and slice. Mix courgettes, beans, peppers and olives adding just enough of the dressing to coat. Leave to cool. Cover and let them sit at room temperature for at least 30 minutes, and up to 2 hours. Taste and adjust seasoning and serve.

Baked Mushrooms with Broad Bean Purée

What is so enjoyable about this combination is the contrast of the rich mealiness of the purée against the smoothness of the baked mushrooms. If it makes life easier, the mushrooms can be grilled instead. The purée is made with Italian Mascarpone cheese – so outrageously calorie-laden that I'd advise you not to scan the label too closely. Still, once in a while . . .

SERVES 4 as a first course
4 large flat cap mushrooms
Olive oil for brushing

For the purée
450 g (1 lb) shelled broad beans
100 g (4 oz) Mascarpone cheese
Squeeze of lemon juice
Salt and freshly ground black pepper

Leaves of 2 sprigs of fresh winter savory
 or fresh thyme
Cayenne pepper

Drop the broad beans into a pan of boiling water. Simmer for 2 minutes, then drain and run the beans under the cold tap. Using a sharp knife, slit the tough outer skin and squeeze out the tender beanlets inside. Discard the skins.

Simmer the skinned beans in salted water until tender – a matter of a couple of minutes. Drain well. Process or liquidize with the Mascarpone and a squeeze of lemon juice. Season with salt and pepper and stir in the savory or thyme. Spoon into a saucepan, ready to be warmed through when needed.

Pre-heat the oven to gas mark 5, 375°F (190°C). Brush the mushrooms with olive oil. Place on a baking sheet, and bake for 20–30 minutes until tender. When they are almost done, re-heat the broad bean purée. Taste and adjust seasonings. Place mushrooms on a dish, and spoon purée on top of them. Dust lightly with cayenne, and serve.

Broad Bean and Goat's Cheese Omelette

This has to be one of the all-time top-league omelettes. A blissful mixture of flavours and once you've skinned and cooked the beans, very little work.

SERVES I
75 g (3 oz) shelled broad beans
3 eggs
1 teaspoon finely chopped fresh dill
Salt and freshly ground black pepper

Butter for frying
25–40 g (1–1½ oz) firm goat's cheese,
 diced

OVERLEAF *Broad Bean and Goat's Cheese Omelette*

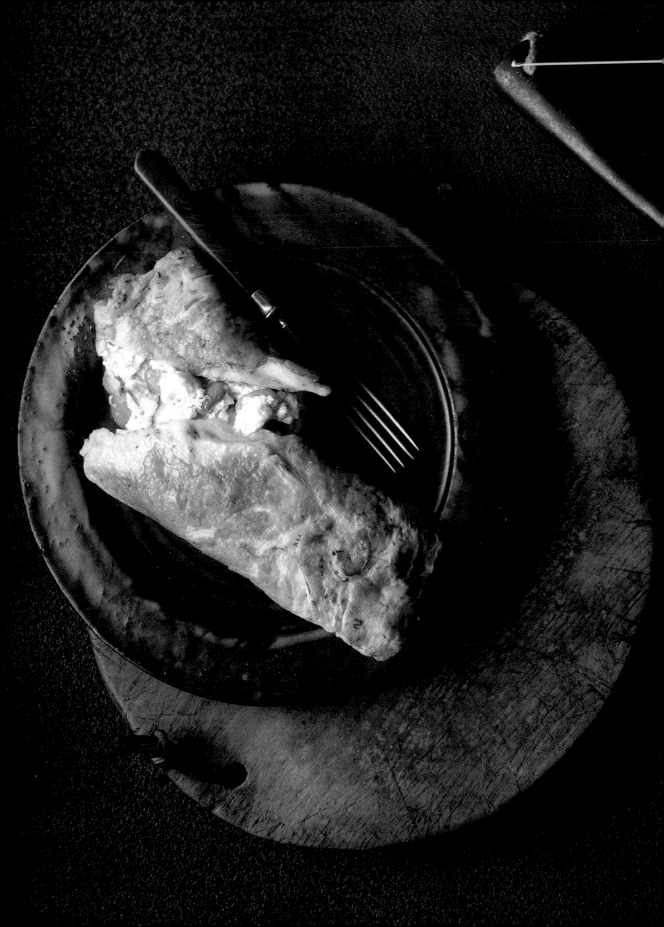

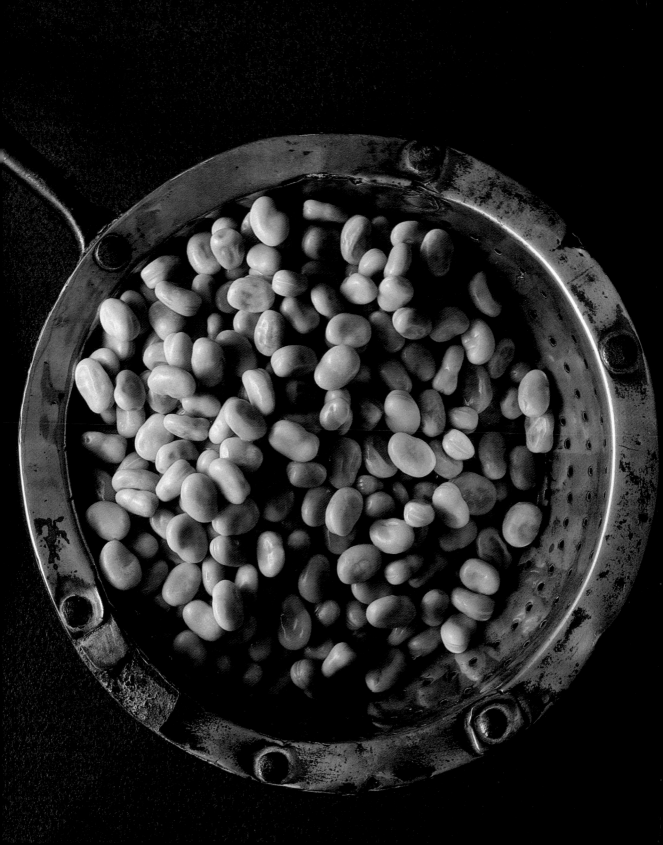

Skip this first part if you are in a hurry or if the beans are very small and tender, but if you have a bit of spare time, it will give you the best possible omelette imaginable. Drop the broad beans into a pan of boiling water. Simmer for 1 minute, then drain and run beans under the cold tap. Using a sharp knife, slit the tough outer skin and squeeze out the tender beanlets inside. Discard the skins.

Simmer the skinned or unskinned beans in salted water until tender – a matter of a couple of minutes for skinned beans, a little longer for unskinned. Drain well.

Beat the eggs, and add the dill, salt and pepper. Melt a knob of butter in a frying-pan and, when it is foaming, pour in the eggs. Scatter the beans over the eggs. Cook, as you would any omelette, scraping in the edges so that the liquid egg can run underneath, until the omelette is set but still moist on the surface. Quickly scatter the goat's cheese over the omelette, roll up, and tip on to a plate. Eat immediately.

Shrimp and Broad Bean Pilau

This is an incredibly delicious pilau, packed with broad beans and shrimps and delicately spiced. It is best, naturally, made with fresh broad beans, though it is not bad made with frozen ones either. To make it really special, blanch and skin the beans before adding them to the rice.

SERVES 4

1 large onion, chopped
2 cloves garlic, peeled and chopped
2 tablespoons sunflower oil
1 teaspoon turmeric
1 teaspoon cumin seeds, bruised with a
   pestle or the end of a rolling-pin
1 teaspoon fennel seeds, bruised
225 g (8 oz) basmati or long-grained
   rice, rinsed

275–450 g (10 oz–1 lb) shelled broad
   beans, thawed if frozen
225 g (8 oz) shelled cooked shrimps
600 ml (1 pint) water
Salt and freshly ground black pepper
2 tablespoons chopped fresh coriander

For the raita
¼ cucumber
Salt
300 ml (10 fl oz) Greek-style yoghurt

First make the raita. Grate the cucumber coarsely without peeling it. Spread it out in a colander and sprinkle with salt. Leave for 30 minutes to 1 hour. Squeeze out excess moisture and then dry on kitchen paper. Mix into the yoghurt and set aside.

In a large saucepan cook the onion and garlic gently in the oil for a couple of minutes. Add the spices and continue cooking until the onion is tender. Stir in the rice and cook for 1 minute longer. Add the water, salt and pepper and bring to the boil. If you are using fresh whole broad beans add these now. Reduce to a simmer, cover tightly and leave to cook for 10 minutes.

Add the shrimps and thawed frozen beans, if using. Stir then cover again and cook for 5–10 minutes until the rice is tender and all the liquid has been absorbed. If necessary add a little more hot water as the pilau cooks. Stir in the coriander, then taste and adjust seasoning. Serve with the cool raita.

Mefarka

Broad beans and mince may not sound too enticing, but add spices, herbs, olive oil and lemon juice and a miracle happens. I found this recipe for Mefarka a few years ago in Claudia Roden's New Book of Middle Eastern Food *(Penguin), and return to it time and again.*

SERVES 6

5 tablespoons light olive oil
450 g (1 lb) shelled broad beans
Salt and freshly ground black pepper
½ teaspoon dried thyme
750 g (1½ lb) lean minced beef
¼ teaspoon freshly ground nutmeg
¼ teaspoon ground cloves

½ level teaspoon cayenne
½ teaspoon cinnamon
3 eggs
Juice of ½ lemon
Chopped fresh parsley
    or coriander to garnish

Mix 3 tablespoons of the oil with 120 ml (4 fl oz) water in a saucepan. Add the broad beans, sprinkle with salt and pepper, and add the thyme. Simmer gently until the beans are tender, adding a little extra water if necessary.

In the meantime, prepare the meat mixture. Heat 2 tablespoons of oil in a deep frying-pan or heavy, flameproof casserole. Add the minced beef when it is just warm – if oil is too hot the meat will dry up. Stir, then add the spices, salt and pepper and just enough water to cover. Simmer until the meat is soft and moist and well-cooked, and has absorbed the water.

Add the meat mixture to the beans and stir well, crushing lightly with a fork. Break the eggs into the pan and stir. Cook, stirring constantly, until they are just set. Turn out on to a serving dish and allow to cool. Taste and adjust seasoning. Serve cold, sprinkled with lemon juice, and parsley or coriander.

Sweetcorn

From the moment sweetcorn is picked, the natural sugars start to convert to starch. Within a couple of hours, the kernels have lost the bulk of their inbuilt sweetness. Sweetcorn growers will usually put the water on to boil before they go to pick the cobs, so that they can get them cooking within 20 minutes while they are still at their peak of perfection.

The race against the ravages of time and nature is something that organic gardener Bob Flowerdew is particularly hot on. His vegetable and fruit garden is one of the most beautiful I've seen, a powerful testament to the efficacy of organic growing methods. It is crammed full of every sort of vegetable and fruit (the raspberries and peaches were sensational), but dominated by stands of sweetcorn. He grows half a dozen different varieties, dotted around the garden so that they don't cross-pollinate. They ripen successively, so that he has a constant supply throughout late summer and early autumn.

We shared some of the first of the year's harvest. The pot of salted water went on the Aga in the chaotic kitchen, and he hurtled out to the garden. Slightly out of breath, he returned five minutes later with two perfect specimens. Off came the husks and the silky threads and, as the bubbles began to rise to the surface, the sweetcorn was ready to slip into the water. We had a sweetcorn feast, butter dripping down our chins as we greedily chewed the honeyed kernels from the cobs. And then we had more – this time grilled rather than boiled, but equally enjoyable.

The trouble with eating sweetcorn as fresh and enticing as that is that you never again want to buy it. Sweetcorn that has been sitting in container lorries and then in storage before finally making it to the sales counter, is old and dull. To be honest you get a better flavour and more sweetness, which is really what sweetcorn is all about, from frozen sweetcorn which will have been rushed from the field to the processing plant with admirable haste.

Sweetcorn and Tomato Salsa

Though the word salsa literally translates as sauce, in the past few years it has come to mean a cold, finely chopped relish, usually made with raw vegetables and fruit, that is served as if it were a sauce proper with grilled fish and poultry. This sweetcorn and tomato salsa is fresh and zippy, and can be made in a couple of shakes. I like to serve it with barbecued chicken. Any left-overs can be stored in the fridge for up to 24 hours. Two heads of sweetcorn will yield about 225 g (8 oz) of kernels.

Preparing Sweetcorn

Whether you grow or buy whole sweetcorn, never keep it hanging around – cook it as soon as possible. If you must store it for a few hours, keep it in the coldest part of the fridge. Don't overcook it. Ten to fifteen minutes in salted boiling water is usually quite long enough.

To cut the kernels from the cobs, stand the cobs upright and slice down close to the tough core, so that the kernels fall off in wide sheets. Scrape the cob over the pan to squeeze out the juice left in the severed bases of the kernels. Add the whole kernels to the pan with a generous knob of butter and salt, cover tightly and cook over a low heat for 5 minutes or so until tender.

Sweetcorn needs a savoury element with it. That may be as simple as butter and coarse sea salt, or a grating of mild cheese. I love it with fried chicken livers – a combination I sometimes use to fill pancakes. The acidity of tomatoes serves well too, maybe in a sauce or diced and mixed with the sweetcorn to make a salsa (see opposite).

SERVES 6

225 g (8 oz) sweetcorn kernels, fresh
  or frozen
350 g (12 oz) ripe tomatoes, skinned,
  de-seeded and finely diced
1–2 fresh green *or* red chillies, de-seeded
  and very finely diced

6 spring onions, sliced very thinly
2 tablespoons chopped fresh coriander
  or fresh basil
Salt and freshly ground black pepper
Juice of ½–1 lime

If you are using fresh corn, put into a saucepan with a tablespoon of water, cover tightly and cook over a low heat for 5 minutes or so until just tender but still slightly crisp. With frozen sweetcorn, just let it thaw. Drain thoroughly, and chop the sweetcorn roughly.

Mix the sweetcorn with all the remaining ingredients, adding lime juice to taste. Cover and leave for at least 1 hour. Stir, taste again and adjust seasoning. Serve at room temperature.

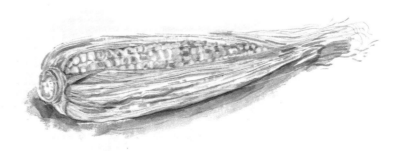

Courgettes Stuffed with Sweetcorn

I came across this recipe in a book called The Cuisines of Mexico *(Harper & Row) by the American food writer, Diana Kennedy, who probably knows more about Mexican cooking than any other non-Mexican. I tried it out, substituting Lancashire cheese for Mexican queso fresco, because it seemed like it would be a good way to use up large courgettes which might otherwise be a touch on the dull side. And so it is . . . turning them into a really stunning dish, far better than you might expect from the simple list of ingredients.*

If you serve the stuffed courgettes as a main course, make a lightly chillied tomato sauce to accompany it (fry a chopped de-seeded chilli or even two, with the onion in the sauce on p. 147).

SERVES 6 as a first course, 4 as a main course

6 plump courgettes, about 750 g (1½ lb) in weight	2 eggs
Salt and freshly ground black pepper	2 tablespoons milk
275 g (10 oz) sweetcorn kernels, thawed if frozen	175 g (8 oz) Lancashire cheese, crumbled
	25 g (1 oz) butter

Cut the courgettes in half lengthwise. Using an apple corer or a sharp-edged teaspoon, scoop out enough of the inner flesh to give a canoe-shaped courgette container, with walls about 1 cm (½ inch) thick. Either save the pulp for another dish, perhaps a soup, or throw it away. Sprinkle the insides of the courgettes lightly with salt and turn upside-down on a wire rack to drain.

Put the corn, eggs, milk and a little salt in a food processor and blend to a knobbly purée. Stir in 100 g (4 oz) of the crumbled cheese and season generously with pepper.

Pre-heat the oven to gas mark 4, 350°F (180°C). Wipe the courgettes dry and set in an oiled ovenproof dish. Fill with the corn mixture. Sprinkle over the remaining cheese and dot with butter. Cover with foil and bake for 30 minutes. Uncover and bake for a further 15–20 minutes until the courgettes are tender and the top lightly browned. Serve hot.

Barbecued Corn-on-the-Cob with Olive and Lemon Butter

Barbecued fresh sweetcorn on the cob, streaked with brown, juicy and tender, has a superb, sweet smoky taste, emphasized by the saltiness of olives in the flavoured butter as it melts over the hot kernels. Soaking the corn plumps up the kernels, ensuring that they don't dry out over the hot charcoal. This is my version of barbecued corn. Alternatively, you could cook them the way Norfolk grower Bob Flowerdew prefers: left in the husk. This method produces a less smoky, more purely sweetcorn flavour. If you choose to leave the husks on, they will still need to be soaked in water for a good 30 minutes. Shake off excess water, then grill over a moderate heat for about 15 minutes, turning frequently.

SERVES 6

6 heads of corn-on-the-cob
Sunflower oil

For the butter

50 g (2 oz) black olives, pitted
100 g (4 oz) unsalted butter, softened
Finely grated zest of ½ lemon

1–2 tablespoons lemon juice
1 small clove garlic, peeled and crushed

Either place all the ingredients for the butter in a food processor and whizz until smooth, or chop the olives very, very finely and mash with the butter and remaining ingedredients. Taste and add extra lemon juice if needed. Pile into a bowl, cover loosely and chill.

Strip the husks and silky threads off the corn. Immerse in a bucket of lightly salted water and leave to soak for at least 30 minutes and up to 3 hours. Just before barbecuing pat dry, brush with oil, then cook over a moderate heat, turning, until patched with brown on all sides. Eat the hot corn with the chilled butter.

My Version of Succotash

Succotash was originally a native American Indian dish of sweetcorn and lima beans thickened with sunflower seed flour. It now appears in almost every general American cookbook. Recipes vary considerably, so I've taken the liberty of doing a bit more tweaking and adapting for myself. Finding lima beans in Britain is not easy (though butter beans bear a close resemblance), so I use green flageolet beans or haricot beans instead. A squeeze or two of lemon juice added right at the end heightens the flavours neatly without making it obviously lemony. And to make it look a little less pallid, as well as adding a touch more taste, I sprinkle chopped parsley on top.

SERVES 6–8

450 g (1 lb) frozen sweetcorn kernels
   or 4 heads of corn-on-the-cob
50 g (2 oz) butter
8 spring onions, cut into
   2.5-cm (1-inch) lengths
Salt and freshly ground black pepper

400 g (14 oz) cooked flageolet
   or haricot beans
150 ml (5 fl oz) double cream
Squeeze of lemon juice
Chopped fresh parsley to garnish

If using fresh sweetcorn, cut the kernels off the cob straight into a saucepan. Scrape down the cob, still over the pan, to extract juices. Put frozen sweetcorn straight into the pan. Add the butter, spring onions, salt and pepper and 4 tablespoons of water. Cover and cook over a low heat for 15 minutes, stirring occasionally. Add the flageolets, or haricots, and cream and simmer, uncovered for 5 minutes or until cream has reduced to a thick sauce. Taste and adjust seasoning, adding a squeeze of lemon juice to bring up the flavour. Sprinkle with a little chopped parsley and serve hot and steaming.

OVERLEAF *Barbecued Corn-on-the-Cob with Olive and Lemon Butter*

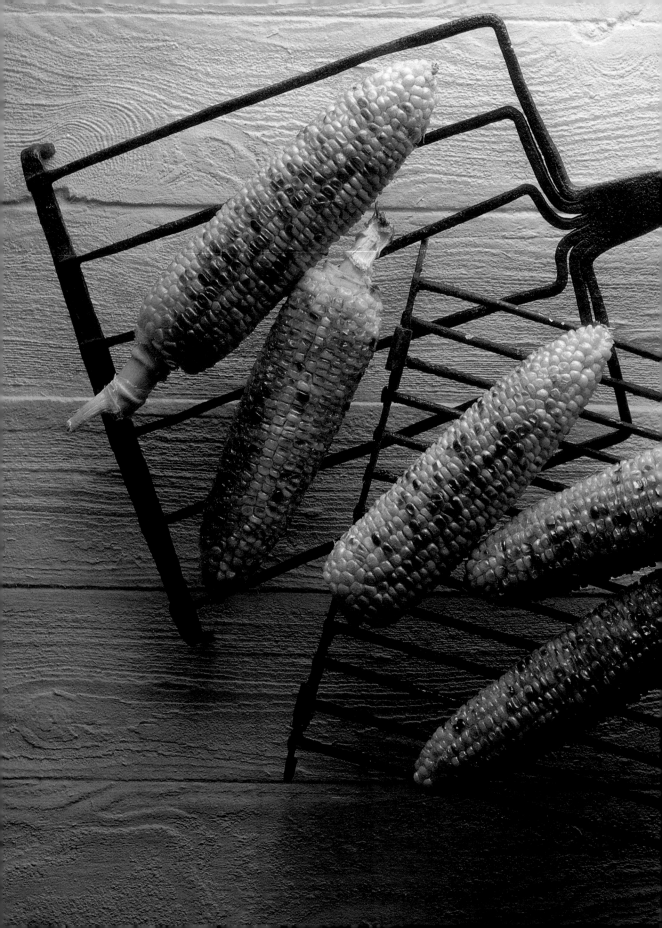

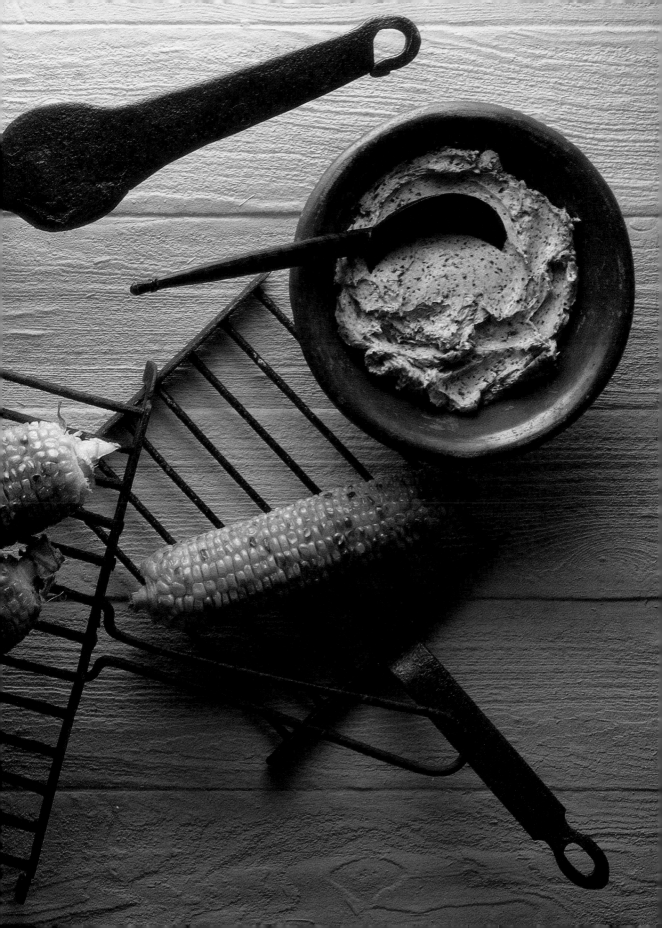

Okra

Okra, bhindi, bamia, ladies' fingers, gumbo – all names for the same, uniquely peculiar vegetable, now a fairly familiar sight in British shops. I'd always imagined that these five-sided, tapering green pods hung down amongst the foliage as they grew. It was a surprise when I saw my first okra plant (not somewhere tropical, but in a greenhouse in north-west England) to discover that they stand erect at an angle to the stem, sturdily pointing towards the skies rather than the earth.

They originated in Africa, travelling up to Egypt, east to India, and carried across the seas by slaves to the Caribbean and southern states of America. Their flavour is delicate and light, much appreciated wherever they are cultivated. What makes them unique, though is their texture, or rather the feel of their juice in the mouth – slippery and viscous. This does not have universal appeal, though for me it is their best characteristic and I would never dream of going out of my way to avoid it.

In some dishes this slippery quality is used to positive advantage, most notably the thick gumbo soup/stews of Louisiana. In soups and sauces, okra gives a marvellous silky smoothness which no one could possibly object to.

Fried Okra

I often use fine cornmeal (from West Indian shops and some supermarkets and delicatessens, but not the same as polenta which is coarsely ground cornmeal) rather than breadcrumbs for coating. It gives the crispest, slightly sweet crust which marries particularly well with the slipperiness of okra. Serve the fried okra as a first course with lemon wedges, or a tomato sauce.

SERVES 4 as a first course

450 g (1 lb) medium-sized okra	Fine cornmeal for coating
Seasoned plain flour for coating	Oil for frying
2 eggs, beaten	Salt and freshly ground black pepper

Trim the okra. Toss in seasoned flour and shake off the excess in a sieve. Tip into the beaten egg, turning carefully to coat, then scoop out, letting excess egg drain off. Finally roll the okra in cornmeal.

Heat a 2.5-cm (1-inch) deep layer of oil in a frying-pan, and fry the okra over a moderate heat, turning once or twice, until evenly browned. Drain briefly on kitchen paper and serve.

Preparing Okra

Although I can't really see the point of trying to remove the one thing that marks okra out from all other vegetables – why buy them in the first place? – there are tricks for dampening down the slipperiness, and I pass them on as a matter of interest. Lemon juice or vinegar is effective. The raw pods can be soaked in well acidulated water for an hour or so, or a dash of lemon juice or vinegar can be added during cooking. Fried okra are less mucilaginous than boiled or steamed. The other trick comes in preparation – trim off the stalk, carefully paring round the conical cap and make sure not to pierce the okra proper. If they are kept whole the juices cannot seep out to lubricate the dish.

When buying okra, choose pods that are on the small side (large ones can be stringy) without brown patches, or at least with as few as possible. They are quite nice eaten raw if small and tender (in which case you may want to scrub them gently under the cold tap to remove the light fuzz) but far better cooked. They can be boiled or steamed whole until just tender – a scant 10 minutes – but it's not the best way to cook them. I prefer them fried gently in butter or oil, sliced or whole. They benefit from the addition of garlic or a few spices, and once cooked a squeeze of lemon or lime juice heightens their flavour. I often simmer them in a tomato sauce, perhaps with fresh coriander, but a new favourite of mine is Bhupinda Samra's Spiced Okra recipe on page 267.

Bamies Yiahni
[Okra in Tomato Sauce]

This Greek-Cypriot way of cooking okra in a tomato sauce is one I particularly like. In Cyprus it may be served as a main course on 'fasting days'. Though it is good hot, I think it is even better cold, with an extra drizzle of olive oil trickled over just before serving.

SERVES 4

450 g (1 lb) okra
3 tablespoons olive oil
1 large onion, chopped
2 cloves garlic, finely chopped
200 g (7 oz) tinned chopped tomatoes

1 tablespoon tomato purée
1 bayleaf
4 tablespoons chopped parsley
Salt and freshly ground pepper

Trim the stalk end off the okra cone without cutting right into the okra. Fry quickly in the oil in a large saucepan, until lightly browned. Spoon into a saucepan.

Fry the onion and garlic in the same oil until tender but without browning. Add the chopped tomatoes and tomato purée, bay leaf and 4 tablespoons water. Bring up to the boil and simmer for 10 minutes. Add plenty of pepper and a pinch of salt. Pour over the okra, then add just enough hot water to cover. Stir in half the parsley. Simmer for 30 minutes, until sauce is thick. Taste and adjust seasonings.

Serve hot or cold, sprinkled with remaining parsley.

Gumbo Ya Ya

Louisiana gumbo is a big soupy stew, but what a stew it is! A classic of Cajun cuisine, there are as many recipes for gumbo as there are cooks who cook it, and probably more. A few things are common to most versions of gumbo (but not all). First the roux, cooked slowly and patiently until it darkens to a deep almost mahogany brown – not just a thickener, but a powerful contributor of flavour. Then there's the 'holy trinity' or in other words, onions, peppers and celery, all chopped finely. And finally, there's okra, or sometimes file *(powdered sassafras). Okra and* file *both give a gumbo its special silky smoothness, but it is only okra that provides flavour as well.*

In Louisiana, gumbo may be served as a first or main course. Either way, it is spooned over a mound of hot rice piled up in individual bowls.

SERVES 6–8 as a main course

120 ml (4 fl oz) sunflower oil	2 green peppers, de-seeded and chopped
1 large chicken, cut into 8 pieces	2 stalks celery, chopped
65 g (2½ oz) plain flour	2 cloves garlic, peeled and chopped
450 g (1 lb) garlic sausage	2 tablespoons finely chopped fresh
or other smoked cooked pork	parsley
sausage, skinned and cut into	1 teaspoon each cayenne pepper and
1-cm (½-inch) slices	black pepper
100 g (4 oz) cooked ham, diced	1 large bay leaf
400 g (14 oz) okra, topped, tailed and	2 sprigs of parsley
halved	2 sprigs of thyme
2 onions, chopped	Salt

In the largest, heaviest flameproof saucepan or casserole you have, heat the oil over a high heat. Brown the chicken pieces evenly in the oil. Set aside. Keep the heat high, and stir the flour into the oil until evenly mixed. Turn the heat down to medium-low and keep stirring with a metal spoon, scraping the brown bits off the base of the pan, until the mixture turns a dark nut brown. (Allow a good 15 minutes or more.)

Then add the sausage, ham, vegetables, garlic and half the parsley. Stir for a minute. Stir in about 150 ml (5 fl oz) water, then add the chicken pieces, both cayenne and black pepper, the bay leaf and sprigs of parsley and thyme tied in a bundle with string, and salt. Gradually add another 1.75 litres (3 pints) of water. Bring to the boil, then simmer for 1 hour, stirring occasionally. Taste and adjust seasonings. Remove the bundle of herbs. Sprinkle with remaining parsley and serve.

Bopinda Samra's Bhindi Sabji
[Spiced Okra]

Bopinda Samra was brought up in Bombay, but her family comes from the Punjab. When she was a child, okra or bhindi, more expensive than other vegetables, was always a great treat. She still cooks it in the traditional Punjab way, with turmeric, ginger, garlic and chillies and just enough tomato to add flavour without dominating the delicate taste of the okra. The method can be adapted to other vegetables, too, though for something like potatoes, say, you will need to add either extra oil or a tablespoon or two of water. She serves 'sabji' with chapattis, or rice, and a wet curry, or dahl.

Garam masala is a mixture of warm aromatic spices, always added at the end of cooking to preserve its fragrance. Bopinda makes her own, but you can buy it ready made in some supermarkets and Indian food shops.

SERVES 4

450 g (1 lb) okra
4 tablespoons sunflower oil
3–4 cloves garlic, peeled and chopped
1½ onions, chopped
1 teaspoon salt
1½ teaspoons grated fresh ginger
1 heaped teaspoon turmeric

1½ thin green chillies, finely chopped
2½ heaped tablespoons chopped tinned
    tomatoes, *or* 2 fresh tomatoes, skinned
    and chopped
1½ teaspoons garam masala (*optional*, but
    a good idea)
A generous squeeze of lemon *or* lime
    juice

Slice the cone and the tip off the okra and discard. Slice okra into 5-mm (¼-inch) lengths.

Heat the oil in a wide frying-pan over a medium to high heat. Add the garlic and fry until beginning to brown, then add the onion and fry until translucent without letting it brown. Next add the salt and mix evenly. Now add the ginger and fry for a few seconds, making sure that it does not stick. Sprinkle over the turmeric and mix, then the chillies. Finally spoon in the chopped tomatoes. Fry for 2–3 minutes, stirring constantly until the tomatoes soften.

Tip in all the okra and stir, scraping residues from the bottom of the pan – the okra will immediately absorb all the oil. Cover and reduce to a low heat. Cook for 15–20 minutes, stirring occasionally, until the okra is tender and the oil is seeping back out. Stir in the garam masala and the lemon or lime juice and serve.

Cornmeal Mush with Okra and Corned Beef

This mush of yellow cornmeal with okra, corned beef and coconut milk is far from elegant in appearance, but I love it. Thick and filling and comforting and packed full of flavour, it is based on Caribbean recipes which explains what at first glance seems an unusual set of ingredients to throw into one pot. Serve it in big steaming dollops, and tuck in.

Coconut milk is not the watery liquid inside a fresh coconut, but a milky juice extracted from the white flesh. You can buy it in tins or frozen, but it is easy to make from desiccated coconut. The same method is used with grated fresh coconut.

Pour 1.2 litres (2 pints) boiling water over 350 g (12 oz) desiccated coconut in a bowl. Stir, and leave until tepid. Strain, squeezing the coconut to extract the milk. Return the coconut to the bowl, and cover with another 600 ml (1 pint) boiling water. Stir and leave again until tepid. Strain, and squeeze coconut hard to extract the last few drops of milk. This makes a fairly thin milk, which is what you need for this recipe.

SERVES 6

1 × 175-g (3-oz) piece unsmoked back bacon, diced
1 tablespoon sunflower oil
1 onion, chopped
225 g (8 oz) tomatoes, skinned and chopped
1–2 fresh red chillies, de-seeded and cut into thin rings
2 sprigs of fresh thyme
 or ½ teaspoon dried

2 tablespoons chopped fresh chives
350 g (12 oz) small okra, trimmed
Salt and freshly ground black pepper
1.5 litres (2½ pints) thin coconut milk
350 g (12 oz) cornmeal or polenta
1 × 350-g (12-oz) tin corned beef, roughly broken into pieces

In a wide heavy saucepan fry the bacon in the oil until lightly browned. Lift out the pieces and reserve. Add the onion, and fry gently until tender, without browning. Now add the bacon, tomatoes, chillies, thyme, 1 tablespoon chives, okra, salt and pepper. Fry, stirring, for 4 minutes.

Stir in coconut milk and bring to the boil. Pour in the cornmeal in a slow steady stream, stirring constantly. Cover and turn the heat right down. Leave to simmer gently for 15 minutes, stirring occasionally, and scraping the bottom of the pan. Add the corned beef, then cover and cook for a further 10 minutes, stirring occasionally. Sprinkle with remaining chives before serving.

Index

Page numbers in *italics* refer to photographs